Risk Profiles in Clinical Nephrology

Contributions to Nephrology

Vol. 37

KARGER

S. Karger · Basel · München · Paris · London · New York · Tokyo · Sydney

2nd European Meeting on Renal Diseases, Milano, February 25–26, 1983

Risk Profiles in Clinical Nephrology

Volume Editor
G. Buccianti, Milano

52 figures and 39 tables, 1984

KARGER

S. Karger · Basel · München · Paris · London · New York · Tokyo · Sydney

Contributions to Nephrology

National Library of Medicine, Cataloging in Publication
European Meeting on Renal Diseases (2nd: 1983: Milan, Italy)
Risk profiles in clinical nephrology/
2nd European Meeting on Renal Diseases, Milano, February 25–26, 1983;
volume editor, G. Buccianti. – Basel; New York: Karger, c1984.
(Contributions to nephrology; v. 37)
Includes index.
1. Hemodialysis – adverse effects – congresses 2. Kidney Diseases – complications – congresses I. Buccianti, G. (Gherardo) II. Title III. Series
W1 CO788UN v. 37 [WJ 300 E895 1983r]
ISBN 3-8055-3739-5

Drug Dosage

The authors and the publisher have exerted every effort to ensure that drug selection and dosage set forth in this text are in accord with current recommendations and practice at the time of publication. However, in view of ongoing research, changes in government regulations, and the constant flow of information relating to drug therapy and drug reactions, the reader is urged to check the package insert for each drug for any change in indications and dosage and for added warnings and precautions. This is particularly important when the recommended agent is a new and/or infrequently employed drug.

Satz: Satzstudio Frohberg, D-6463 Freigericht
Printed in Switzerland by Thür AG Offsetdruck, Pratteln
ISBN 3-8055-3739-5

Contents

Round Table Discussion:

Can Long-Term Complications Resulting From Dialytic Treatment Be Prevented Through Suitable Treatment of Chronic Renal Insufficiency?

Haemodialysis and Membrane Biocompatibility

Round Table Discussion:

Substantive Parameters Involved in Blood Membrane Biocompatibility

Prediction of Renal Risk in Pregnancy

Foreword

The Second European Meeting on Renal Diseases was held in Milan in February 1983, in accordance with the decision of the Milan Association for the Prevention and Therapy of Renal Diseases to organize an International Scientific Meeting every other year with the object of examining some of the most debated topics in the field of nephrology. The present volume, a result of the meeting, affords a profile of the recent progress achieved in all the topics examined.

It now seems well established that renal stone disease – especially when calcium stone formation is concerned – depends on a balance between promoter and inhibitor factors. The papers presented at the session 'Risk profiles in renal stone formation' deal with the role of environmental, dietary, socioeconomic and urinary risk factors in the genesis of urinary calculi. Moreover, one of the most important points was to determine the exact role of hypercalciuria in the laboratory assessment of stone-former patients and to emphasize the emerging concept that a defect in renal tubular function might be one of the main factors leading to stone formation.

The round table 'Can long-term complications resulting from dialytic treatment be prevented through suitable treatment of chronic failure?' was conceived to make the point regarding the actual possibilities of decreasing the rate of progression of renal failure through dietary restriction and better control of hypertension.

Another point to examine was the protective effect of more timely control of hypertension upon cardiovascular risk in order to establish if the accelerated atherosclerosis seen in uremic patients correlates with the rate of progression of hypertension or with the duration of dialytic treatment.

The papers presented in that session also dealt with the main problem related to the control of secondary hyperparathyroidism, especially in the early stage of chronic renal failure. The scope of the session regarding hemodialysis and membrane biocompatibility was to seek a better definition of biocompatibility and to examine the substantial parameters involved in order to establish an international standardized test in the near future.

Improvement of hemodialysis techniques in recent years allowed a longer survival of the patients, but emphasized in some of them symptoms such as pruritus, fatigue and pulmonary dysfunction.

It is therefore always increasingly necessary that manufacturers of hemodialysis membranes stress not only the characteristics of permeability, surface and clearance of the various molecules, but also the features of better biocompatibility.

Last but not least, 'Prediction of renal risk in pregnancy' deals with the clinical prospects of the outcome of pregnancy for the mother and the offsprings in the course of renal disease, whether the disorder involves glomerular or tubulointerstitial tissue. Restoration of normal renal and endocrine functions by means of renal transplant allows the patients to become pregnant and to achieve a successful outcome in more than half of the cases considered.

The meeting would not have been a success without the valuable support of the Scientific Committee and of the sponsors to whom I wish to express my gratitude.

Gherardo Buccianti, Istituto di Clinica Medica 1°, Servizio di Nefrologia e Dialisi, Università di Milano, Italia

Contr. Nephrol., vol. 37, pp. 1–4 (Karger, Basel 1984)

Metabolic and Biochemical Risk Factors in Renal Stone Disease

W.G. Robertson, M. Peacock

MRC Mineral Metabolism Unit, The General Infirmary, Leeds, UK

The simplest model of urinary stone disease describes it as being due to periods of excessive crystalluria. This may be so great or persistent that crystal aggregates form and become lodged at some narrow section of the urinary tract and there form the nucleus of a stone. The formation of abnormal crystals and aggregates is dependent on the degree of supersaturation of urine with the salt concerned and the balance between the levels of inhibitors and promoters of crystallisation in urine. The so-called 'abnormalities' in urine leading to increased supersaturation and decreased protection by inhibitors may be referred to as *urinary risk factors*. These 'abnormalities', in turn, are secondary to various environmental and metabolic factors which can be thought of as *pre-urinary risk factors for the disorder* (table I).

Cystine Stones

Cystine stone disease is the simplest form of the disorder to account for. This only occurs in patients who are homozygous for a rare autosomal recessive disease characterised by a defect in the tubular reabsorption of cystine which is relatively insoluble in urine. Above a urinary concentration of 1,250 μmol/l cystine crystalluria and stone formation occur. Homozygous cystinurics generally have urinary cystine concentrations in excess of this value. Heterozygotes, on the other hand, have concentrations below the critical value and do not form stones. Normal subjects excrete even lower concentrations of cystine.

Table I. Risk factors for the various types of urinary stone formation

Type of stone former	% Occurrence	Composition	'Pre-urinary' risk factors	Main urinary risk factors
Cystine	1–3	cystine	inherited defect in amino acid transport	↑ cystine
Uric acid	4–16	uric acid	renal ammonia production; ileostomy	↓ pH
			gout; ↑ purine intake; glycogen storage disease; Lesch-Nyhan syndrome; neoplastic disease	↑ uric acid
			percutaneous loss of fluid; diarrhoea; ileostomy	↓ volume
Infection	7–31	calcium phosphate + magnesium ammonium phosphate	urinary tract infection with urea-splitting organism	↑ ammonia; ↑ pH
Calcium	58–81	calcium oxalate and/or calcium phosphate	age and sex	↑ calcium, ↑ oxalate, ↑ uric acid, ↑ pH, ↓ ABPP inhibitors, ↓ volume
			climate; season	↓ volume, ↑ calcium, ↑ oxalate
			fluid intake	↓ volume
			affluence and diet	↑ calcium, ↑ oxalate, ↑ uric acid
			metabolic disorders:	
			primary hyperparathyroidism	↑ calcium, ↑ pH, (?) ↑ oxalate
			renal tubular acidosis	↑ pH, ↑ calcium
			hyperoxaluria	↑ oxalate

Uric Acid Stones

Such a simple clear-cut separation, however, does not exist between stone formers and controls for other forms of stone disease. In the case of uric acid stones, two factors are of importance in determining the risk of crystalluria, namely, the concentration of uric acid and the acidity of urine (table I). Most normal urines are undersaturated or within the metastable region of supersaturation with respect to uric acid. In contrast, patients with uric acid stones have significantly higher supersaturation levels usually above the point of spontaneous precipitation of uric acid. Crystalluria is a common finding in this group. The pre-urinary risk factors leading to these 'abnormalities' are presented in table I.

Infection Stones

Stones formed secondary to urinary tract infection are composed of magnesium ammonium phosphate with variable amounts of calcium phosphate. These occur more commonly in women than in men and onset often dates from pregnancy. The *Proteus* group of gram-negative bacteria and certain coliform bacteria are the most common causes of this type of stone. They possess the enzyme urease which breaks down urea to ammonia and produces a very alkaline urine. These are the major risk factors for the disorder (table I).

Calcium Stones

Of all the stone-forming salts, calcium oxalate and calcium phosphate are potentially the most insoluble under the ionic conditions present in urine. Indeed, the supersaturation of urine with respect to calcium oxalate is very close to the point of spontaneous precipitation even in normal urine. This probably accounts for these salts being the most common constituents of urinary stones.

The urinary risk factors for calcium stone disease are more complex than those responsible for other stone types (table I). The controlling factor is the balance between the level of supersaturation (determined largely by volume, pH and the excretions of calcium and oxalate) and the net level of inhibitory activity (dependent mainly on the urinary concentrations of alcian blue precipitable polyanions (ABPP) and urate).

In only a few instances does any one of the above urinary risk factors account for stone disese in a given individual. In the vast majority of patients, the disorder appears to be *multifactorial*, resulting from a combination of changes (sometimes small) in the excretion of two or more urinary risk factors. By combining all six measurements, it is possible to assess the risk of forming calcium-containing stones in a given individual.

W.G. Robertson, MD, Medical Research Council, Mineral Metabolism Unit,
The General Infirmary, Great George Street, Leeds LS1 3EX (England)

Contr. Nephrol., vol. 37, pp. 5–8 (Karger, Basel 1984)

The Role of Glycosaminoglycans and Uric Acid in Idiopathic Calcium Nephrolithiasis

B. Baggio, G. Gambaro, A. Marchi, E. Cicerello, S. Favaro, A. Borsatti

Clinica Medica I, Università di Padova, Italia

Introduction

Recent clinical and experimental studies sustain a pathogenetic role of uric acid in calcium oxalate (CaOx) renal stone disease [1–3]. To establish a relationship between uric acid and CaOx, two hypotheses have been advanced. The first one theorises the possibility that urate crystals promote epitaxic CaOx crystallization [4, 5], whereas the second proposes that uric acid or sodium urate remove some yet undefined mucopolysaccharides (GAGs), which on their own exert an inhibitory action on CaOx crystal growth and aggregation [6–9]. In fact, an interaction between uric acid and some GAGs, such as heparin and chondroitin sulfate has been demonstrated in artificial solutions [7–9], but this effect has never been observed in whole urine.

The purpose of this study was to verify whether a bond between GAGs and uric acid could be demonstrated in whole urine. To this end, GAGs excretion was evaluated in 3 groups of patients with different urine uric acid levels.

Patients and Methods

Patients

(1) 22 control subjects; (2) 24 recurrent idiopathic calcium oxalate renal stone formers; (3) 21 patients with biopsy confirmed glomerulonephritis; (4) 15 insulin-dependent diabetics in good metabolic control with no proteinuria. Patients and controls all had sterile urines, and normal renal function as assessed by creatinine clearance.

Table I. Urinary values (mean ± SD) of pH, uric acid, GAGs and U/UF_1 ratio in controls (C), stone formers (SF), glomerulonephritics (GN) and diabetics (D)

	C	SF	GN	D	F	p<
pH	6.12 ± 0.38	6.10 ± 0.37	6.15 ± 0.40	6.11 ± 0.42	0.08	n.s.
Uric acid, mg/g creatinine	120.78 ± 53.97	265.20 ± 174.49	227.43 ± 120.68	702.00 ± 303.75	35.36	0.01
GAGs mg/g creatinine	43.34 ± 16.61	32.68 ± 14.75	63.43 ± 28.14	98.14 ± 72.00	11.85	0.01
U/UF_1	1.39 ± 0.34	2.58 ± 2.22	1.82 ± 0.81	8.29 ± 4.00	36.75	0.01

Methods

Urine was collected from 7 to 9 a.m., centrifuged at 2,000*g* for 10min, and filtered through a 0.22-µm (Millipore) filter. A sample of the filtered urine was used for the determination of pH, uric acid [10], GAGs [11] and creatinine. Uric acid and GAGs excretion was expressed per gram creatinine. A further urine sample was filtered in an Amicon apparatus with a UM2 filter. Uric acid concentration was evaluated before (U) and after ultrafiltration (UF_1), and the results expressed as the ratio U/UF_1. In order to evaluate a possible surface effect of the membranes, 10 urine samples underwent a second ultrafiltration through the same apparatus using the same filter size and the ratio UF_1/UF_2 was recorded.

Statistical evaluation was carried out using analysis of variance (one-way) and the coefficient 'r' of correlation.

Results

Mean values of pH, uric acid, GAGs, and the U/UF_1 ratio found in patients and controls are reported in table I. No significant difference in urine pH ($F = 0.08$) emerged. Urine GAGs excretion was significantly different in the 4 groups ($F = 11.85$; $p < 0.01$), as well as urinary uric acid and the U/UF_1 ratio ($F = 35.36$; $p < 0.01$; $F = 36.75$; $p < 0.01$).

A statistically significant direct correlation was found between total urine uric acid concentration and the ratio U/UF_1 ($r = 0.86$; $p < 0.001$). No correlation was found between GAGs urinary excretion and the U/UF_1 ratio ($r = 0.18$).

Reultrafiltration did not promote any significant loss of uric acid (UF_1/UF_2 ratio: $t = 0.26$), thus excluding an aspecific membrane surface effect.

Discussion

The main result emerging from this study is the demonstration of non-ultrafiltrable uric acid in the urine of the patients studied, which correlated well with uric acid concentration. Since a membrane surface effect was excluded, uric acid non-ultrafiltrability may be explained by the following mechanisms: (a) The existence of a bond between uric acid and some urinary mucopolysaccharides, as first suggested by *Robertson* [6]; (b) the existence of a bond between uric acid and other unidentified substances present in the urine; and (c) the existence of uric acid in a colloidal form in urine.

The first hypothesis was advanced [6] in an attempt to explain the 'facilitating action' exerted by uric acid on calcium oxalate renal stone disease, but it was demonstrated only in vitro in simple solutions and not in whole urine [7–9]. If non-ultrafiltrable uric acid were only due to a bond with GAGs, it follows that we should have found a direct relationship between GAGs and non-ultrafiltrable uric acid concentration, but we were unable to find such a correlation.

The presence of non-ultrafiltrable uric acid in urine might, however, well be due to a yet unidentified substance(s) different from GAGs, but capable of binding uric acid. While we have no data to exclude this possibility, it seems unfeasible since we found a direct relationship between total uric acid and non-ultrafiltrable uric acid concentrations. It follows that if this substance(s) is present, its excretion should parallel that of uric acid, which is improbable, albeit possible.

We consider the third possibility, i.e., the existence of uric acid in a colloidal form in urine, the most feasible, and this view is strengthened by the demonstration of a direct relationship between the uric acid and non-ultrafiltrable uric acid concentration. In an attempt to extrapolate from our data the influence uric acid might have in promoting CaOx stone formation, two further consideration should be made. Regarding the hypothesis that uric acid favors CaOx stone formation by binding and removing some GAGs present in the urine, such reducing of their inhibitory activity, is not supported by our findings. If colloid uric acid is important per se in promoting the epitactic growth of CaOx crystals, it must be taken in serious account that the non-ultrafiltrable uric acid found in a population of renal stone formers was not higher than in other pathological conditions, such as diabetes and glomerulonephritis, and it seem to follow the same physicochemical law.

Finally, the possible existence of a bond between uric acid and other high molecular weight substances different from GAGs deserves further studies.

References

1 Coe, F.L.; Kavalach, A.G.: Hypercalciuria and hyperuricosuria in patients with calcium nephrolithiasis. New Engl. J. Med. *291*: 1344–1350 (1974).

2 Coe, F.L.: Treated and untreated recurrent calcium nephrolithiasis in patients with idiopathic hypercalciuria, hyperuricosuria or no metabolic disorder. Ann. intern. Med. *87*: 404–410 (1977).

3 Pak, C.Y.C.; Waters, O.; Arnold, L.; Holt, K.; Cox, C.; Barilla, D.: Mechanism for calcium urolithiasis among patients with hyperuricosuria. J. clin. Invest. *59*: 426–431 (1977).

4 Coe, F.L.; Lawton, R.L.; Goldstein, R.B.; Terube, V.: Sodium urate accelerates precipitation of calcium oxalate in vitro. Proc. Soc. exp. Biol. Med. *149*: 926–929 (1975).

5 Pak, C.Y.C.; Arnold, L.H.: Heterogenous nucleation of calcium oxalate by seeds of monosodium urate. Proc. Soc. exp. Biol. Med. *149*: 930–932 (1975).

6 Robertson, W.G.: Physical-chemical aspects of calcium stone-formation in the urinary tract; in Fleisch, Robertson, Smith, Vahlensieck, Urolithiasis research, pp. 25–39 (Plenum Press, New York 1976).

7 Finlayson, B.; Du Bois L.: Adsorption of heparin on sodium acid urate. Clinica chim. Acta *84*: 203–206 (1978).

8 Pak, C.Y.C.; Holt, K.; Zerwekh, J.E.: Attenuation by monosodium urate of the inhibitory effect of glycosaminoglycans on calcium oxalate nucleation. Investive Urol. *17*: 138–140 (1979).

9 Baggio, B.; Gambaro, G.; De Nardo, L.; Borsatti, A.: The role played by acid mucopolysaccharides in calcium oxalate nephrolithiasis (Abstract). Kidney int. *22*: 95 (1982).

10 Liddle, L.; Seegmiller, J.E.; Laster, L.: The enzymatic spectrophotometric method for determination of uric acid. J. Lab. clin. Med. *54*: 903–913 (1959).

11 Whiteman, P.; Henderson, H.: A method for the determination of amniotic-fluid glycosaminoglycans and its application to the prenatal diagnosis of Hurler and Sanfilippo diseases. Clinica chim. Acta *79*: 99–105 (1977).

Bruno Baggio, MD, Clinica Medica I, Policlinico Universitario, I-35100 Padova (Italy)

Contr. Nephrol., vol. 37, pp. 9–12 (Karger, Basel 1984)

Environmental Factors in the Development of Urolithiasis

Sverker Ljunghall

Department of Internal Medicine, University Hospital, Uppsala, Sweden

Principally stone formation of the urinary tract should be divided into two parts – upper and lower urinary tract stones. Bladder stones have for many centuries occured endemically in Europe and Asia, and still do in less developed countries. Epidemiological studies [1] have presented strong evidence that dietary factors are of great importance in this context. With an increasing consumption of animal protein, bladder stone formation ceases to be an nationwide problem. The mechanisms responsible for this association have however not been completely revealed.

Kidney and ureteric calculi, on the other hand, appear to be increasingly common in the industrialized part of the world. At our own hospital the admission rates for stones have increased more than tenfold over the last part of this century [2]. Similar increases have been reported in a number of studies. Since this changing pattern of stone formation has occurred during a period when there have been enormous changes in general life-style, it is natural that the question arises if there are causal associations between environmental factors and stone formation.

In order to establish such a direct relationship ideally, studies should be designed where individuals were randomized to controlled changes of the environment and followed prospectively over several years. No such investigations appear to have been performed. The second best might be to analyze in detailed cross-sectional and longitudinal studies differences in stone disease between well-defined populations. However, it is then important to realize that stone symptoms are largely managed outside the hospital and that any study that ignores outpatients will seriously underestimate the incidence rates [2]. The extent to which hospital admission rates (which are much easier to obtain) reflect the true incidences depends, for example, on access to and policies for inpatient care.

There are great differences in the pattern of stone disease between the western industrialized countries on one hand, and that reported from e.g. Brazil, Sudan and Thailand. The available data do not permit even an attempt to analyze which factors that are of greatest importance for these differences. Large *geographical variations* have been reported for the prevalence of renal stone disease also within the industrialized world [3, 4]. However, in studies where evaluations have been made of the unselected population a fairly similar picture emerges. About 10% of the males and 3–5% of the females will have developed at least one stone by the age of 60 with the peak incidence occurring around the age of 40. Each year 0,5–1% of the male population will experience symptoms of a stone. The differences between the different studies from Scandinavia [2], FRG [5], Great Britain [6] and USA [7] are not greater than they can largely be explained by different methodological approaches. This would exclude at least very important local environmental factors that are not shared by the studied populations.

It has been claimed that *climate* plays some role with stones in many reports being more common during the warm period of the year. This might be due to increased exposure to sunlight with the ensuing raised production of vitamin D in the skin, hypercalciuria and hyperoxaluria appearing as consequences [9].

The hardness of *drinking water* might be of some importance. Hospital admission rates in the United States were inversely related to the water content of calcium and magnesium [3, 10]. Similar reports have for example come from Great Britain and Finland. Such a relationship, which at first seems paradoxical, could be due to an increased binding of oxalate in the intestine, an increased solubility of urinary calcium oxalate or to other, unknown, factors. However, a correlation has not been evident in all studies. Possibly the use of private wells and domestic water softeners have been confounding factors.

Dietary habits, in particular the probable negative influence of an increased consumption of animal protein, have been extensively discussed [11, 12]. An association has been demonstrated at four different demographic levels between an increased consumption of animal protein and the hospital admission rates for renal stone [11]. However, a controlled dietary study could not detect any differences between the diets of renal stone formers and matched controls [13]. Thus, it has not yet been proven that consumption of animal protein fulfills all criteria for an epidemiological risk factor. Also other food constituents have been implicated such as carbohydrates, fat, fiber and alcohol but not verified to be of causal importance.

A dramatic change in life-style which has developed during the last century is the models of *occupation*. As regards formation of renal stones very few studies have tried to analyze if occupational hazards could be of importance. In a recent investigation from Scotland it was found [14] that coppersmiths, who are chronically exposed to cadmium, have a markedly increased propensity to form stones. Few other occupations have been studied as thoroughly. In general terms it seems as if laborers have a lower incidence of stones compared to white-collar workers [2], but if this is related to the occupation or only reflects the different socioeconomic factors has not been evaluated.

Short-term exposure to physical or psychological *stress* [15] will raise the urinary calcium excretion. It has also been reported that the urinary output of protective factors such as magnesium and citrate will be reduced [15]. The relevance of these experiments for our daily life has not been determined.

In conclusion, there is no doubt that there has been a changing pattern in stone formation of the urinary tract during the 20th century. It seems likely that environmental factors that have appeared during this time are of importance. However, with few exceptions these potentially harmful factors in our environment have not been proven guilty with reasonable certainty. The many suggestions that have been proposed should be followed up with controlled studies before therapy and prevention of stones can be adjusted accordingly.

References

1 Andersen, D.A.: The nutritional significance of bladder stones. Br. J. Urol. *34*: 160–177 (1962).

2 Ljunghall, S.: Renal stone disease – studies of epidemiology and calcium metabolism. Scand. J. Urol. Nephrol. *41*: suppl., pp. 1–96 (1977).

3 Boyce, W.H.; Garvey, F.K.; Strawcutter, H.E.: Incidence of urinary calculi among patients in general hospitals, 1948 to 1952. J. Am. med. Ass. *161*: 1437–1442 (1956).

4 Nordin, B.E.C.; Hodgkinson, A.: Urolithiasis. Adv. internal Med. *13*: 155–182 (1967).

5 Tschöpe W.; Ritz, E.; Haslbeck, M.; Mahnert, H.; Wesch, H.: Prevalence and incidence of renal stone disease in a German population sample. Klin. Wschr. *59*: 411–412 (1981).

6 Scott, R.; Freeland, R.; Mowat, W., et al.: The prevalence of calcified upper urinary tract stone disease in a random population – Cumbernauld health survey. Br. J. Urol. *49*: 589–595 (1977).
7 Johnson, C.M.; Wilson, D.M.; O'Fallon, W.M.; Malek, R.S.; Kurland, L.T.: Renal stone epidemiology: a 25-year study in Rochester, Minnesota. Kidney int. *16*: 624–631 (1979).
8 Hiatt, R.A.; Dales, L.G.; Friedman, G.D.; Hunkeler, E.M.: Frequency of urolithiasis in a prepaid medical care program. Am. J. Epidem. *115*: 255–265 (1982).
9 Elomaa, I.; Karonen, S.-L.; Kairento, A.-L.; Pelkonen, R.: Seasonal variation of urinary calcium and oxalate excretion, serum 25(OH)D_3 and albumin level in relation to renal stone formation. Fortschr. Urol. Nephrol. *17*: 121–126 (1982).
10 Churchill, D.; Bryant, D.; Fodor, G.; Gault, M.H.: Drinking water hardness and urolithiasis. Ann. intern. Med. *88*: 513–514 (1978).
11 Robertson, W.G.; Peacock, M.: Heyburn, P.J.; Speed, K.; Hanes, F.: The role of affluence and diet in the genesis of calcium-containing stones. Fortschr. Urol. nephrol. *11*: 5–14 (1978).
12 Robertson, W.G.; Peacock, M.: The pattern of urinary stone disease in the United Kingdom in relation to animal protein intake during the period 1960–1980. Urol. int. *37*: 393–399 (1982).
13 Griffith, H.M.; O'Shea, B.; Kevany, J.P.; McCormick, J.S.: A control study of dietary factors in renal stone formation. Br. J. Urol. *53*: 416–420 (1981).
14 Scott, R.F.; Cunningham, C.; McLelland, A.; Fell, G.S.; Finch, O.P.; McKellan, N.: The importance of cadmium as a factor in calcified upper urinary tract stone disease – a prospective 7-year study. Br. J. Urol. *54*: 584–589 (1982).
15 Brunding, P.; Berg, W.; Schneider, H.-J.: Stress and Harnsteinbildungsrisiko. Urol. int. *36*: 199–207, 265–273 (1981).

S. Ljunghall, MD, Department of Internal Medicine, University Hospital, S-75185 Uppsala (Sweden).

Contr. Nephrol., vol. 37, pp. 13–16 (Karger, Basel 1984)

Pathophysiology and Signification of Hypercalciuria in Calcium Stone Formers

André Ulmann

Départment de Physiologie, Hôpital Necker, Paris, France

Among other metabolic abnormalities, hypercalciuria constitutes a risk factor for calcium stone formation [1]. Therefore, search for increased urinary calcium excretion is commonly undertaken in renal stone formers (SF). Further, drugs that decrease urinary calcium output are sometimes prescribed to decrease the risk of new stone formation. However, the pathophysiology and the predictive value for stone recurrence of high urinary calcium excretion is unclear in many respects. It is also of interest to determine if diet-induced modifications of calciuria can explain, at least in part, why the frequency of stone disease has significantly risen during the last 30 years [2].

The purpose of the 3 different studies reported here was twofold: (1) to investigate the effect of glucose on calciuria, and to determine the relationship between calcium and sodium excretion in normal and in stone-forming subjects; and (2) to look for a possible predictive value of hypercalciuria for the recurrence of stone formation.

Patients and Methods

In the first study, we investigated 17 SF with idiopathic hypercalciuria (IH), i.e. calciuria above 7mmol/day for men and 6mmol/day for women, 6 normocalciuric (NC) SF, and 10 normal subjects. After an overnight fast, they were given 100g glucose orally. 30-min urine collections were performed immediately and 30 and 60min after glucose ingestion. Plasma was sampled in the middle of each urine collection. Calcium, glucose and creatinine were measured in each plasma and urine sample.

In the second study, 24-hour urine collections were performed each day during a 3-day hospitalization in 21 normal subjects, 62 IHSF and 36 NCSF. The mean of daily calcium, sodium, uric acid and oxalate excretion was taken into account. The SF were retrospectively

Table I. Plasma glucose (PG) and urinary UCa/creat. before and after glucose ingestion

	Fasting	After glucose	
		30 min	60 min
PG, mmol/l			
Controls	4.4 ± 0.2	6.8 ± 0.7***	6.0 ± 0.9*
IH SF	4.4 ± 0.1	8.5 ± 0.6**	6.8 ± 0.9**
NC SF	4.3 ± 0.2	7.8 ± 0.8***	6.8 ± 0.9*
UCa/creat., mmol/mmol			
controls	0.22 ± 0.03	0.37 ± 0.06*	0.46 ± 0.06
IH SF	0.42 ± 0.05	0.57 ± 0.06***	0.74 ± 0.07
NC SF	0.24 ± 0.04	0.49 ± 0.09	0.62 ± 0.11*

*$p<0.05$; **$p<0.01$; ***$p<0.001$ vs. fasting value.

classified has having a 'severe' or a 'benign' stone disease: 'severe' lithiasis was defined as de novo formation of 3 stones or of 1 staghorn calculus in the preceding 5 years.

In the third study, urinary calcium excretion was determined in 38 SF before and during treatment with high water intake alone (19 patients), or in combination with thiazide administration (hydrochlorothiazide, 50 mg once daily). The stone recurrence rate was defined as the number of new stones actually formed divided by the number of years spent either since the first stone was discovered (pretreatment stone recurrence rate) or since treatment was initiated (on-treatment stone recurrence rate).

In all studies, plasma and urine calcium was determined by atomic absorption, oxalate by gas chromatography and other parameters by standard automated procedures.

Results and Discussion

The influence of glucose ingestion on urinary calcium excretion is reported in table I. In the 3 groups a significant increase in urinary calcium to creatinine ratio (UCa/creat.) was found after glucose ingestion. In addition, a significant overall positive correlation was found between weight index and both fasting UCa/creat. ($r=0.36$, $p<0.05$) and the maximal increase in UCa/creat. after glucose ingestion ($r=0.42$, $p<0.02$). The results indicate that urinary calcium excretion is, at least partially, dependent upon weight in normal and stone-forming subjects. Plasma glucose tended to be higher in IHSF whose weight index was significantly higher than that of normal subjects and of NCSF. Therefore, hypercalciuria in IHSF is in part

Table II. 24-hour urinary excretion of calcium, oxalate and uric acid in SF with 'severe' or 'benign' urolithiasis (mean ± SD)

	Calcium mmol/day	Oxalate mmol/day	Uric acid mmol/day
Severe lithiasis	5.8 ± 2.3	211 ± 115	3.9 ± 1.1
Benign lithiasis	6.6 ± 2.9	217 ± 134	3.6 ± 1.2

related to some degree of glucose intolerance that probably results from overweight.

When measured during a 3-day hospitalization while on a controlled diet (1 g calcium and phosphorus daily) daily sodium as well as calcium excretion was higher in IHSF than in control or NCSF. Further, a positive linear correlation was found in IHSF as in normal subjects between urinary sodium and creatinine, but the slope of the regression line was significantly higher in IHSF than in controls (IHSF: Na = 7.2 creat. + 14.8; Na = 3.8 creat. + 10.9; $p < 0.001$ between slopes). Similarly, a positive linear correlation was found between calcium and creatinine both in IHSF and controls. The slopes of the regression lines also differed significantly between the 2 groups ($p < 0.001$). These findings are evidence for abnormal calcium and sodium handling in IHSF leading to higher Na and Ca excretion per mole of creatinine than in control subjects. No such relations were found in NCSF, probably because this group is heterogeneous and comprises patients resembling IHSF with tubular disturbances and patients with no tubular abnormalities. The results of these studies are in good agreement with results from previously reported studies [3]. Thus, high urinary calcium output in SF appears, at least in part, dependent upon glucose ingestion and is associated with elevated sodium excretion.

Whatever its pathophysiology, it is of importance to look for a predictive value of hypercalciuria for the recurrence of stone formation. Patients studied while on a 3-day hospitalization were classified as having a 'severe' or a 'benign' lithiasis as indicated in the Patients and Methods section. Table II indicates the mean 24-hour values for calcium, oxalate and uric acid in the 2 groups. No difference was apparent between values found in the 2 groups. Further, 'severe' lithiasis was not more frequent in subjects with urinary excretion of calcium and/or oxalate and/or uric acid above the mean ±2 SD values found for all SF.

In the study performed in patients prescribed a high water intake alone or in combination with thiazide therapy, pretreatment stone recurrence rate (0.72 and 0.88 stones/year, respectively) was unrelated to the magnitude of 24-hour urinary calcium excretion. In the patients given thiazides, a transient decrease in urinary calcium excretion was noted 1 year after initiation of thiazide but was not found later. Meanwhile, a significant decrease in stone recurrence rate occurred in both groups (to 0.30 and 0.24 stones/year, respectively) that was unrelated to the variations of urinary calcium excretion. Although the dosage of thiazide was lower than that usually recommended [4], it was efficient since a slight but significant rise in plasma calcium was noted in thiazide-treated patients.

In conclusion, pathophysiological investigations indicate that hypercalciuria in SF is at least partially related to dietary glucose and is associated with impairment of tubular sodium handling. Our data also indicate that the importance of daily urinary calcium excretion is by itself unrelated to the severity of the disease in terms of new stone formation and is of no value for predicting stone recurrence.

References

1 Nordin, B.E.C.: Hypercalciuria. Clin. Sci. mol. Med. *52*: 1–8 (1977).

2 Johnson, C.M.; Wilson, D.M.; O'Fallon, W.M.; Malek, R.S.; Kurland, L.T.: Renal stone epidemiology: a 25-year study in Rochester, Minnesota. Kidney int. *16*: 624–631 (1979).

3 Sutton, R.A.L.; Walker, V.R.: Responses to hydrochlorothiazide and acetazolamide in patients with calcium stones: evidence suggesting a defect in renal tubular function. New Engl. J. Med. *302*: 709–713 (1980).

4 Yendt, E.R.; Cohanim, M.: Prevention of calcium stones with thiazides. Kidney int. *13*: 397–409 (1978).

A. Ulmann, MD, Département de Physiologie, Hôpital Necker, 161 rue de Sèvres, F-75730 Paris Cédex 15 (France)

Contr. Nephrol., vol. 37, pp. 17–21 (Karger, Basel 1984)

Increased Probability of Forming Stones with a Simple Calcium Restriction in Idiopathic Hypercalciuria

P. Bataille[a], *J. Gregoire*[a], *G. Charransol*[b], *A. Pruna*[a], *B. Coevoet*[a], *A. Fournier*

[a]Service de Néphrologie, CHU Amiens, France; [b]Institut d'Hydrologie, CHU Pitié Salpétrière, Paris, France

A low calcium diet is the usual therapeutic advice given to any stone formers without taking into account the pathophysiological basis of their disease or their usual dietary intake of oxalate. An appreciable decrease in calciuria can be achieved by a low calcium diet but this measure induces a rise in oxalate excretion [1, 2]. This increase of renal excretion of oxalate could be explained by the increase of the passive oxalate absorption by the colon since decreasing the calcium load in the intestinal lumen will increase the concentration of free oxalate anions available for absorption. However, some findings do not support this scheme: *Barilla* et al. [3] found a comparable increase of oxaluria after oxalate load in absorptive and renal hypercalciuria as in controls, and for *Galosy* et al. [4] urinary oxalate excretion was not significantly different in stone formers with absorptive hypercalciuria [5] when the diet was changed from a random to a calcium-restricted diet. Because of these controversies, it seemed to us justified to study the effect of dietary calcium restriction on the renal excretion of oxalate and calcium in controls and ambulatory stone formers maintained on a free oxalate diet, and to evaluate the resultant effect of their expected opposite changes by the changes of 'the probability of being a stone former' (PSF) [6].

Patients and Methods

50 healthy controls and 51 patients with calcium urolithiasis were studied on an ambulatory protocol. They collected their 24-hour urines while on a free diet and after 3 days of calcium restriction without oxalate restriction. On day 5 at 7 a.m. they drank 300ml of distilled water, whereas they were fasting since 8 p.m. on the day before and collected their 2-hour fasting urine and had blood samples drawn. At 9 a.m. they took 1g of calcium orally and at 1 p.m. urine and blood were again collected. On all urine samples, creatinine, calcium, phosphate and sodium were measured. Oxalate was measured only on the two 24-hour urine collections. Before and after the oral calcium load, blood samples were analyzed for calcium, phosphate, creatinine, protein and C- and N-terminal parathyroid hormone (PTH).

Calcium, phosphate and creatinine were determined by automatic colorimetry (Technicon autoanalyzer) and oxalic acid by gas-liquid chromatography. PTH was measured by C- and N-terminal specific radioimmunoassay. Statistical differences were assessed by the Student's t test.

Results

Classification of Patients

17 patients were normocalciuric, and 34 patients were hypercalciuric on unrestricted diet (calciuria > normal + 2SD, i.e. > 380mg/day in men and 280mg(day in women). They were classified according to *Pak* et al. [5], but with our own controls data, into the following groups:

– Absorptive hypercalciuria type 1 (AH1) was defined by increased calciuria on free and calcium-restricted diet, a normal fasting urinary calcium/urinary creatinine (UCa/UCr) ratio (< 0.12 in men and < 0.13 in women) and normal plasma PTH levels. This type represents the classic presentation with high intrinsic intestinal absorption.

– Absorptive hypercalciuria type 2 (AH2), which is due to excess intake of calcium, is defined by hypercalciuria on an unrestricted diet and normal calciuria on a restricted diet comparatively to controls on a restricted diet (calciuria < normal + 2SD, i.e. < 280mg/day in men and 180mg/day in women). Their fasting UCa/UCr ratio is normal as well as the plasma PTH levels.

– Renal hypercalciuria (RH) due to a primary renal leak of calcium is characterized by increased calciuria on both free and calcium-restricted diets, an elevated fasting UCa/UCr ratio and high subsequently suppressed PTH levels with calcium load.

– Primary hyperparathyroidism was found in 3 patients who presented hypercalciuria on days 2 and 4, increased fasting UCa/UCr ratio, hypercalcemia and nonsuppressive PTH levels.

Table I. Daily urinary excretion of calcium and oxalate (mean ± SEM) before and after calcium restriction, and the changes of the PSF with calcium restriction (CaR)

Patients groups and controls	Calciuria, mg/day		Oxaluria, mg/day		PSF changes with
	before CaR	after CaR	before CaR	after CaR	CaR
Controls (n = 50)	195 ± 9	120 ± 7**	29 ± 1	34 ± 1*	+0.01
Normocalciuria (n = 17)	210 ± 16	150 ± 10**	38 ± 2	44 ± 2.5*	−0.02
Absorption calciuria type 2 (n = 11)	433 ± 30	193 ± 10***	35 ± 4	45 ± 6*	−0.23**
Absorption calciuria type 1 (n = 10)	378 ± 26	289 ± 15**	40 ± 2	55 ± 4**	+0.07*
Renal calciuria (n = 10)	383 ± 50	365 ± 49**	34 ± 3	45 ± 4**	+0.10*

Significance of the difference between before and after calcium restriction: *$p<0.05$; **$p<0.01$; ***$p<0.001$.

Effect of a Low Calcium Diet on the Renal Excretion of Calcium and Oxalate in Controls and Patients

Table I shows the values of daily UCa and oxalate excretions before and after calcium restriction in controls and stone formers. In all groups, there was a significant decrease of calciuria and a significant increase of oxaluria.

The comparison of stone formers with the controls show that calciuria is of course greater in the hypercalciuric groups, but the decrease of calciuria with calcium restriction is significantly greater than that observed in controls only in the group AH2 ($p<0.001$). Oxaluria before and after calcium restriction is greater in all groups of stone formers. The increase of oxaluria with calcium restriction is greater than in controls only for the stone formers with AH1 ($p<0.01$) or RH ($P<0.05$) but not for the stone formers with normocalciuria or AH2.

Determination of the Probability of Being a Stone Former (PSF) and Variations of the PSF with Calcium-Restricted Diet

The PSF was determined by the method of *Robertson* et al. [6] with the use of our own control and patient data. The frequency distribution curves of the 24-hour excretion of calcium and oxalate and the risk curves for oxaluria and calciuric determined by the ratio (α) of the (frequency of stone formers)/(frequency of normals) at each value of oxaluria and calciuria have been published elsewhere [7]. The PSF combining the risk factors Ca and Ox was calculated by using the equation:

$$\mathrm{PSF} = \frac{\alpha\mathrm{Ca} \cdot \alpha\mathrm{Ox}}{1 + \alpha\mathrm{Ca} \cdot \alpha\mathrm{Ox}} .$$

It was then possible to determine for each patient the PSF on a free diet and on a restricted diet and then to evaluate the effect of the calcium restriction.

Discussion

Our study has shown the following points: (1) stone formers have usually higher excretion of calcium and oxalate than controls on both diets; (2) calcium restriction induces a decrease in calcium excretion and an increase in oxalate excretion without a change in urine output in all groups; (3) the importance of the changes varies greatly with the underlying pathophysiology: calciuria decreased more markedly in AH2 due to usual excessive calcium intake and oxaluria increased more markedly in AH1 and RH, i.e. the 2 varieties of idiopathic hypercalciuria.

The resulting probability of being a stone former was unchanged in the controls and in the patients with normocalciuria. It decreased significantly only in AH2, whereas it increased significantly in AH1 and RH.

Our findings are in full agreement with those of others [1, 2, 8] as regards the dependency of oxalate excretion on the state of calcium absorption and intake. These data are opposite to those of *Galosy* et al. [4] who, in long-term ambulatory study, could not find any significant increase in oxaluria when a calcium-restricted diet is recommended. However, this discrepancy could be explained by the fact that their patients were already on a low oxalate diet. Therefore, the following operating scheme can be proposed: oxalate excretion changes is critically dependent on the passive absorption of oxalate by the colon. This latter is dependent upon the availability of free oxalate and therefore on the intake of oxalate and on the amount of calcium escaping more proximal intestinal absorption. This explains why the increase of oxalate excretion with calcium restriction is more pronounced on a high oxalate diet, and at a constant oxalate intake when intestinal calcium absorption is truly increased, as in idiopathic hypercalciuria.

From a practical point of view, a low calcium diet appears to be beneficial only in the patients with dietary hypercalciuria. For the other patients these results suggest that simultaneous restriction of oxalate intake should be added to calcium restriction. The real efficiency of this double dietary restriction on the PSF as well as its practicability remain to be evaluated.

References

1 Zarembski, P.M.; Hodgkinson, A.: Some factors influencing the urinary excretion of oxalic acid in man. Clinica chim. Acta *25*: 1–10 (1969).

2 Marshall, B.W.; Cochran, M.; Hodgkinson, A.: Relationships between calcium and oxalic acid intake in the diet and their excretion in the urine of normal and renal stone forming subjects. Clin. Sci. *43*: 91–99 (1972).

3 Barilla, D.E.; Notz, G.; Kennedy, D.; Pak, C.Y.C.: Renal oxalate excretion following oral oxalate loads in patients with ileal disease and with renal and absorptive hypercalciuria. Effect of calcium and magnesium. Am. J. Med. *64*: 579–585 (1978).

4 Galosy, R.; Clarke, L.; Ward, D.L.; Pak, C.Y.C.: Renal oxalate excretion in calcium urolithiasis. J. Urol. *123*: 320–323 (1980).

5 Pak, C.Y.C.; Britten, F.; Peterson, R.; Ward, D.; Northcatt, C.; Breislaun, A.; MacGuire Sakhar, K.; Busch, S.; Nicar, M.; Normand, A.; Peter, S.P.: Ambulatory evaluation of nephrolithiasis classification, clinical presentation and diagnostic criteria. Am. J. Med. *69*: 19–30 (1980).

6 Robertson, W.G.; Peacock, M.; Heyburn, P.J.; Marshall, D.H.; Clark, P.B.: Risk factors in calcium stone disease of the urinary tract. Br. J. Urol. *50*: 449–454 (1978).

7 Bataille, P.; Charransol, G.; Gregoire, I.; Fournier, A.: Effect of calcium restriction on renal excretion of oxalate and the probability of forming stone in the various pathophysiological groups of calcium stone formers. J. Urol. (in press, 1983).

8 Hodgkinson, A.: Evidence of increased oxalate absorption in patients with calcium-containing renal stones. Clin. Sci. mol. Med. *54*: 291–294 (1978).

Prof. A. Fournier, Service de Néphrologie, Hôpital Nord, F-80000 Amiens (France)

Contr. Nephrol., vol. 37, pp. 22–26 (Karger, Basel 1984)

Effects of Low Calcium Diet on Urinary Calcium and Oxalate Excretion in Patients with Idiopathic Calcium Nephrolithiasis

Giacomo Colussi[a], *Antonio Antonacci*[a], *Maurizio Surian*[b], *Giuseppe Pontoriero*[a], *Giuseppe Rombolà*[a], *Maria Elisabetta De Ferrari*[a], *Pablo Cosci*[b], *Fabio Malberti*[b], *Luigi Minetti*[a]

Renal Units, [a]E.O. Niguarda Ca' Granda-Milan, and [b]Ospedale Maggiore-Lodi, Milan, Italy

Hypercalciuria is a common finding in patients with idiopathic calcium (Ca-oxalate and/or Ca-phosphate) stone disease, and a widely recognised risk factor of this kind of nephrolithiasis [1]. However, the role of Ca as an important factor responsible for urine oversaturation has been a matter of debate. On the one hand, the fall in urinary CaOx saturation (evaluated as APR or CPR) following the reduction of Ca excretion with thiazide [2, 3], sodium cellulose phosphate [3] or orthophosphate [3, 4] suggests an important pathogenetic role of hypercalciuria per se in Ca stone formation; on the other hand, it has been suggested that Ca plays only a modest role in urinary saturation for calcium oxalate (CaOx), whereas a much greater effect is exercised by Ox [5]. As a consequence, 'mild' hyperoxaluria (as frequently observed in Ca stone formers), would be much more important than hypercalciuria in increasing urinary saturation for CaOx and the risk of stone formation [6].

Dietary Ca restriction is highly effective in reducing Ca excretion in most patients with idiopathic hypercalciuria [7]; since, however, a low Ca diet increases intestinal absorption and urinary excretion of Ox, unless Ox intake is also reduced [8], this therapeutic approach has been claimed to be theoretically contraindicated in Ca stone formers [6]. In a study on outpatients, Ox excretion was unaffected by changes in Ca intake [9], suggesting that Ca restriction does not necessarily increase Ox excretion.

The present study was undertaken to verify the changes in urinary Ca and Ox excretion, and in CaOx urine saturation, following low Ca diet in a group of 'idiopathic' CaOx stone formers, classified according to different metabolic profiles in relation to Ca excretion.

Patients and Methods

64 out-patient 'idiopathic' CaOx stone formers (43 males and 21 females), aged 18–53 years, and 10 healthy controls (6 males and 4 females, aged 21–46 years), underwent two 24-hour urine collections at the end of a 10-day period of either 1 g (normal) or $<$400 mg (low) Ca diet. Caloric, salt, protein and Ox content was kept free, but high-Ox-containing foods were forbidden: calculated Ox content of the diets was in the low-normal range of 0.7–1.3 mmol (60–120 mg), and did not change significantly on the two Ca regimens. The patients were classified according to their Ca excretion (UCaV) on either diet: in normocalciuric (NC) patients UCaV was less than 8 (♂) and 7 (♀) mmol/day (320 and 280 mg/day) on 1 g Ca diet, and less than 7.5 (♂) and 6.5 (♀) mmol/day (300 and 260 mg/day) on low Ca diet. These values are the upper 95% confidence limits in our healthy population. Diet-dependent (DD) hypercalciuric patients had high UCaV on 1 g Ca diet, but normal UCaV on low Ca diet; diet-independent (DI) hypercalciuric patients had high UCaV on either diet. Urines, collected with thymol and mineral oil, were analyzed for Ca (atomic absorption spectrophotometry) and Ox [10]. Urinary saturation with respect to CaOx was evaluated in relation to the thermodynamic solubility product of CaOx (relative supersaturation, RS) and expressed in log units [11]. Statistical analysis was performed by use of paired and unpaired Student's t test, as indicated.

Results

Ca and Ox excretion, urine volume and urine RS on the two diets are shown in table I. RS was not different between most stone formers and controls despite high UCaV and UOxV in DD and DI, due to higher urine output in the patients. UCaV fell on low Ca diet in controls and DD, but the changes in UOxV were not significant. As a result, urine RS significantly fell in DD, and remained unchanged in the other groups. After correction of individual RS values for a standard urine volume, the fall of RS in DD was still significant ($p<0.05$). Multiple linear regression analysis disclosed significant correlations between RS and urine volume in NC ($r=-0.79$ and -0.77 on either diet, $p<0.001$), and DD ($r=-0.65$ and -0.75, $p<0.001$); between RS and Ox concentration in controls ($r=0.92$, $p<0.001$, and 0.82, $p<0.01$), NC ($r=0.82$ and 0.9, $p<0.001$), DI ($r=0.95$ and 0.91, $p<0.001$) and DD ($r=0.91$ and 0.84, $p<0.001$); between RS and Ca concentration only in NC on either diet ($r=0.69$ and 0.81, $p<0.001$), in controls on 1 g Ca diet ($r=0.63$, $p<0.05$), whereas in DD

Table I. Urinary Ca (UCaV), oxalate (UOxV) and volume (vol), and CaOx relative supersaturation (RS) on normal (1 g) and low (<400 mg) Ca diet in normal controls and CaOx stone formers

	1 g Ca diet				< 400 mg Ca diet			
	UCaV, mmol/day	UOxV, mmol/day	vol, liters	log RS	UCaV, mmol/day	UOxV, mmol/day	vol, liters	log RS
Controls (n = 10)	5.06± 1.85	0.35± 0.14	1.22± 0.24	1.00± 0.14	3.51± 1.45**	0.46± 0.12	1.33± 0.13	1.03± 0.09
NC (n = 30)	5.08± 1.57	0.40± 0.16	1.85± 1.08	0.94± 0.20	4.07± 1.42	0.45± 0.17	2.14± 0.77	0.88± 0.21
DI (n = 11)	11.52 3.07	0.59± 0.28	2.07± 0.53	1.05± 0.14	9.80± 2.21	0.60± 0.19	2.24 0.77	1.04± 0.08
DD (n = 23)	9.69± 2.32	0.54± 0.20	1.86± 0.96	1.09± 0.12	5.11± 1.61*	0.62± 0.28	2.06± 1.39	0.99± 0.16**
Controls vs. NC	NS	NS	p < 0.01	NS	NS	NS	p < 0.001	p < 0.005
Controls vs. DI	p < 0.001	p < 0.025	p < 0.001	NS	p < 0.001	NS	p < 0.001	NS
Controls vs. DD	p < 0.001	p < 0.005	p < 0.005	NS	p < 0.01	p < 0.05	p < 0.02	NS

vs. 1 g Ca diet, *p<0.001; **p<0.01 (paired t test).

the correlation was better ($r = 0.74$, $p < 0.001$) on low than on normal ($r = 0.59$, $p < 0.01$) Ca diet.

In figure 1, it is shown that in all patients, RS was better correlated with Ca concentration on low than on normal Ca diet: at low Ca concentrations (less than 3 m*M*), the relationship between Ca and RS was very steep, so that the less the Ca concentration, the less the urine RS.

Discussion

The results of this study show that low Ca diet is able to reduce in many Ca stone formers UCaV without any consistent uncrease in UOxV. When

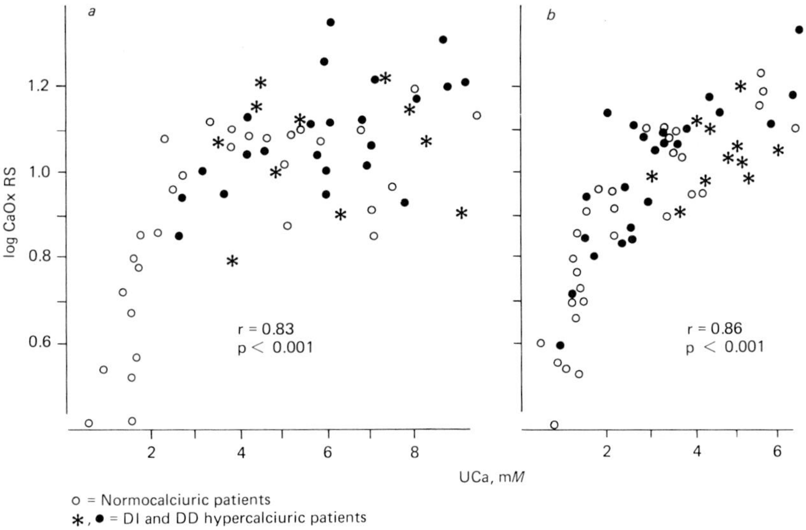

Fig. 1. Relationship between Ca concentration (UCa) and urine relative supersaturation (RS). *a* 1 g Ca diet. *b* <400 mg Ca diet.

Ca restriction was able to significantly reduce urinary Ca excretion and concentration, a fall in urine CaOx RS ensued: the less the Ca concentration on the low Ca diet, the less the urine CaOx RS, independently of the presence or absence of hypercalciuria on 1 g Ca diet (fig. 1). Thus, Ca excretion after a low Ca diet is the main parameter to select those patients for whom Ca restriction might be indicated. We deliberately chose to give no special advice on diet composition except for its Ca content and with the avoidance of a few high-oxalate foods, since dietary approach to stone disease, a lifelong treatment, must be simple to be well accepted and really followed.

These data do not lessen the importance of the influence of Ox in urine CaOx saturation; indeed in all the groups CaOx RS was highly correlated with Ox concentration on either diet, and hypercalciuric patients had evidence of the so-called 'mild hyperoxaluria' [6] on both diets. Any reduction in its urinary excretion would be predicted to induce very consistent effects on the state of urine saturation. Unfortunately, dietary Ox restriction is much less effective in reducing urinary excretion than Ca restriction. The validity of our saturation parameters resides in the validity of the method we used [11]: it is a simplification of a more complete one [5], with which it has compared well [11]. However, similar results to ours were obtained with the more complete method by *Marshall* et al. [8] in 8 stone formers, of which 2 were normocalciuric and 6 DD hypercalciuric, according to our definition. That study showed also that the effects of low Ca diet could be much potentiated by parallel oxalate restriction.

References

1 Robertson, W.G.; Peacock, M.; Heyburn, P.J.; Marshall, D.M.; Clark, P.B.: Risk factors in calcium stone disease of the urinary tract. Br. J. Urol. *50*: 449–454 (1978).

2 Weber, D.V.; Coe, F.L.; Parks, J.H.; Dunn, M.S.; Tembe, V.: Urinary saturation measurements in calcium nephrolithiasis. Ann. intern. Med. *90*: 180–184 (1979).

3 Pak, C.Y.C.; Galosy, R.A.: Propensity for spontaneous nucleation of calcium oxalate. Am. J. Med. *69*: 681–689 (1980).

4 Pak, C.Y.C.; Holt, K.; Zerwekh, J.; Barilla, D.: Effects of orthophosphate therapy on the cristallisation of calcium salts in urine. Mineral Electrolyte Metab. *1*: 147–154 (1978).

5 Robertson, W.G.; Nordin, B.E.C.: Activity products in urine; in Hodgkinson, Nordin, Renal stone research symposium, pp. 221–232 (Churchill Livingstone, London 1969).

6 Robertson, W.G.; Peacock, M.: The cause of idiopathic calcium stone disease: hypercalciuria or hyperoxaluria? Nephron *26*: 105–110 (1980).

7 Lemann, J.: Idiopathic hypercalciuria; in Coe, Brenner, Stein, Nephrolithiasis, pp. 86–115 (Churchill Livingstone, New York, 1980).

8 Marshall, R.W.; Cochran, M.; Hodgkinson, A.: Relationship between calcium and oxalic acid intake in the diet and their excretion in the urine of normal and renal stone-forming subjects. Clin. Sci. *43*: 91–99 (1972).

9 Galosy, R.W.; Clarke, L.; Ward, D.L.; Pak, C.Y.C.: Renal oxalate excretion in calcium urolithiasis. J. Urol. *123*: 320–323 (1980).

10 Hodgkinson, A.; Williams, A.: An improved colorimetric procedure for urine oxalate. Clinica chim. Acta *36*: 127–132 (1972).

11 Marshall, R.W.; Robertson, W.G.: Normograms for the estimation of the saturation of urine with calcium oxalate, calcium phosphate, magnesium ammonium phosphate, uric acid, sodium acid urate, ammonium acid urate and cystine. Clinica chim. Acta *72*: 253–260 (1976).

G. Colussi, MD, Renal Unit, E.O. Niguarda Ca'–Granda-Milan,
Piazza Ospedale Maggiore 3, I-20162 Milan (Italy)

Contr. Nephrol., vol. 37, pp. 27–30 (Karger, Basel 1984)

Urinary Composition and Supersaturation on a High Protein Diet

Bengt Fellström[a], Bo G. Danielson[a], Britta Karlström[b], Hans Lithell[b], Sverker Ljunghall[a], Bengt Vessby[b]

Departments of [a]Internal Medicine and [b]Geriatrics, University Hospital, Uppsala, Sweden

Introduction

A dietary intake of purine-rich animal protein has been claimed to be the basis for an increased incidence of urolithiasis in the western world [1]. The urinary excretion of calcium and oxalate has been reported to increase with dietary animal protein [2]. Urinary urate was also related to the amount of purines or proteins in the diets [2, 3]. The object of the present investigation was to further elucidate the metabolic effects of a high dietary intake of animal protein, and concomitant effects on urinary composition and supersaturation.

Material and Methods

8 calcium stone patients were admitted to a metabolic ward for 4 weeks and fed on a low protein diet (LPD) for 2 weeks and on a high protein diet (HPD) for 2 weeks. The two diets were isoenergetic, contained equal amounts of fat and the difference in the protein calories was balanced by carbohydrates. The LPD contained 12 % protein and 48 % carbohydrates, whereas the HPD contained 29 % protein and 31 % carbohydrates. The amount of protein in LPD was 57 g/2,000 kcal and in HPD 142 g/2,000 kcal. The excess of protein in HPD was mainly animal protein. The two diets contained equal amounts of calcium and oxalate. There were no restrictions regarding the fluid intake.

By the end of each dietary period, the urinary excretion of electrolytes, organic acids and nitrogen compounds were measured. Urine pH was measured on freshly voided urine in the morning. Calcium and magnesium were analyzed by atomic absoprtion, urate and citrate enzymatically and oxalate colorimetrically. Supersaturations, ionic activities and urinary complexes were calculated through solving the thermodynamic mass equations by using an iterative, computerized procedure (Equil) [4].

Table I. 24-Hour excretion of urinary constituents (mean ± SD) on low protein (LPD) and high protein (HPD) diets

	LPD	HPD	p
Urine volume, ml	1,717 ± 597	1,973 ± 459	n.s.
Calcium, mmol	5.55 ± 1.85	7.43 ± 2.71	$p < 0.02$
Phosphate, mmol	26.0 ± 5.6	42.9 ± 8.8	$p < 0.001$
Magnesium, mmol	4.43 ± 0.89	4.75 ± 1.08	n.s.
Citrate, mmol	4.3 ± 1.5	3.1 ± 1.2	$p < 0.001$
Oxalate, mmol	0.35 ± 0.04	0.37 ± 0.06	n.s.
Sulphate, mmol	14.2 ± 1.3	39.6 ± 7.1	$p < 0.001$

Results

The 24-hour excretion of calcium increased in all subjects (table I), 70% of the increase being in the night portion. Urinary phosphate also increased whereas urinary magnesium did not differ on the two diets. Urinary citrate decreased on the HPD whereas urinary oxalate was unchanged.

There was a 90% increase in urinary urate from 3.5 ± 0.4 to 6.6 ± 1.0 mmol/24h ($p < 0.001$) and increased excretion of both titratable acid and ammonium ions on HPD compared with LPD ($p < 0.001$). The morning urine pH was 0.9 pH units lower ($p < 0.05$) on HPD compared with LPD.

The calculated ion activity product (AP) of calcium oxalate was within the metastable limits on both diets and the net effect on calcium oxalate supersaturation was not different on HPD compared with LPD. On the other hand, the ion activity product of uric acid increased in all patients. The urines were all undersaturated on LPD but supersaturated in 5 patients on HPD. The ion activity product of ammonium urate was within the metastable region on both diets, but a higher degree of supersaturation was seen on HPD (fig. 1). The sodium urate ion activity product was not different on the two diets.

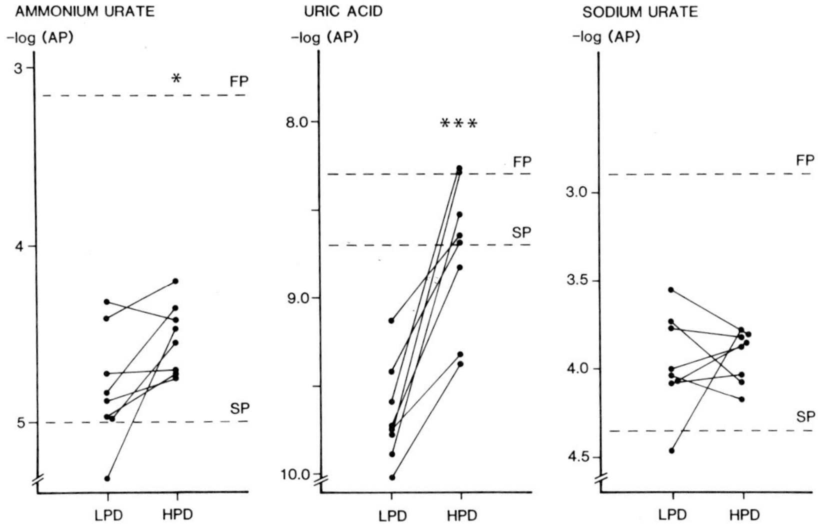

Fig. 1. Ion activity products of ammonium urate, uric acid and sodium urate on low protein (LPD) and high protein (HPD) diets. FP = Formation product; SP = solubility product. $^{*}p<0.05$; $^{***}p<0.001$.

Discussion

In the present investigation, just like in previous studies, urinary calcium and urate became increased on purine-rich animal protein diet [2, 3]. The reason for the induction of calciuria on HPD is believed to be a primary renal effect and not an increased intestinal absorption [5]. The mechanism is probably a decreased tubular reabsorption of calcium complexes. This view is supported by the fact that the urinary excretion of cyclic AMP was higher on HPD than on LPD (not shown).

Dietary purines become absorbed in the intestine and further metabolized to urate, which is subsequently mainly excreted in the urine [6]. Because of a high content of ash acids in proteins the urinary content of titratable acid and ammonium ions increased profoundly on HPD, and there was also a drop in the urine pH. Urinary citrate was in the high-normal range on the LPD but decreased by 27% on HPD. The degree of acidity probably stimulated the renal oxidation of citrate and caused a diminished excretion.

The propensity for crystal formation, growth and aggregation depends on the balance between urinary supersaturation and inhibitory activity.

The net effect on calcium oxalate supersaturation was not different on the two diets by the current method. On the other hand, the risk of forming uric acid or ammonium urate crystals or stones was significantly higher on HPD than on LPD. Microcrystals of uric acid are weak promoters of calcium oxalate crystallization [7] but may also under certain conditions interfere with naturally occurring macromolecular inhibitors of calcium oxalate crystal growth [8]. Furthermore, the decrease in urinary citrate and pH on HPD may have an unfavorable effect on the inhibitory activity of calcium oxalate crystal growth.

It is concluded that the risk of forming uric acid or ammonium urate crystals or stones becomes increased on a high protein diet. Calcium oxalate supersaturation, on the other hand, is not different on the two diets but the inhibitory activity of calcium oxalate crystal growth and aggregation may become affected unfavorably.

References

1 Robertson, W.G.; Peacock, M.; Heyburn, P.J.; Hanes, F.; Swaminathan, R.: The risk of calcium stone formation in relation to affluence and dietary animal protein; in Brockis, Finlayson, Urinary calculus, pp. 3–12 (PSG Publishing Company, 1981).

2 Robertson, W.G.; Heyburn, P.J.; Peacock, M.; Hanes, F.A.; Swaminathan, R.: The effects of high animal protein intake on the risk of calcium stone formation in the urinary tract. Clin. Sci. *57*: 285–288 (1979).

3 Coe, F.L.; Moran, E.; Kavalach, A.G.: The contribution of dietary purine overconsumption to hyperuricosuria in calcium oxalate stone formers. J. chron. Dis. *29*: 793–800 (1976).

4 Finlayson, B.: Calcium stones: some physical and clinical aspects; in David, Calcium metabolism in renal failure and nephrolithiasis, pp. 337–382 (Wiley, Chichester 1977).

5 Allen, L.H.; Bartlett, R.S.; Block, G.D.: Reduction of renal calcium reabsorption in man by consumption of dietary protein. J. Nutr. *109*: 1345–1350 (1979).

6 Löffler, W.; Gröbner, W.; Zöllner, N.: Influence of dietary protein on serum and urinary uric acid; in Rapado, Watts, de Bruyn, Purine metabolism in man. III, vol. 122A, pp. 209–214 (Plenum Press, New York 1979).

7 Pak, C.Y.C.; Arnold, L.H.: Heterogenous nucleation of calcium oxalate by seeds of monosodium urate. Proc. Soc. exp. Biol. Med. *149*: 930–932 (1975).

8 Fellström, B.; Backman, U.; Danielson, B.G.; Holmgren, K.; Ljunghall, S.; Wikström, B.: Inhibitory activity of human urine on calcium oxalate crystal growth: effects of sodium urate and uric acid. Clin. Sci. *62*: 509–514 (1982).

B. Fellström, MD, Department of Internal Medicine, University Hospital, S-75185 Uppsala (Sweden)

Contr. Nephrol., vol. 37, pp. 31–35 (Karger, Basel 1984)

Immobilization: A Cause of Resorptive Hypercalciuria

A. Jeantet, G. Giachino, P. Rossi, C. Tetta, A. Thea, G. Squiccimarro, V. Calitri, A. Vercellone

Cattedra di Nefrologia dell'Università, Divisioni di Nefrologia e Dialisi, Ospedale Maggiore S.G. Battista; Istituto di Clinica Ortopedica I dell'Università, Torino, Italia

Introduction

Although immobilization has been known for many years to cause hypercalciuria and, sometimes, hypercalcemia as well as the skeletal features so-called 'disuse osteoporosis', the pathogenetic mechanisms responsible for these alterations are still controversial. Recent pathophysiologic studies have suggested that immobilization-induced hypercalciuria may be consequent to a resorptive pathogenesis associated with depression of the parathyroid hormone (PTH)$-1,25(OH)_2D3$ axis [3]. In this paper, the alterations of mineral metabolism and their sequence were investigated in order to suggest a pharmacologic approach to specific treatment of bone resorption and urolithiasis prevention in prolongedly immobilized patients.

Materials and Methods

We selected 27 patients (21 M, 6 F; age: 37.3 ± 15.1 years; duration of immobilization: 51.9 ± 29.7 days, mean $\pm$ 1 SD). The cause of immobilization were fractures (77.7%), hip dislocation (11.1%), coxarthrosis (7.4%) and scoliosis (3.7%). The frequency of surgery was 44%. No past history of renal and/or urological pathology was present. Renal function was normal in all patients (BCrC = 138.8 ± 49.7 ml/min). Our protocol comprised studies on serum (creatinine – Cr; calcium – Ca; phosphorus – P; magnesium – Mg; PTH; alkaline phosphatase – APh), on urine (fasting U_{Ca}/U_{Cr}, U_{OHPr}/U_{Cr} as in [2]), finally on renal phosphorus threshold [4] and on Mg excretion index (MgEI). All statistical studies were performed using the Student's t test.

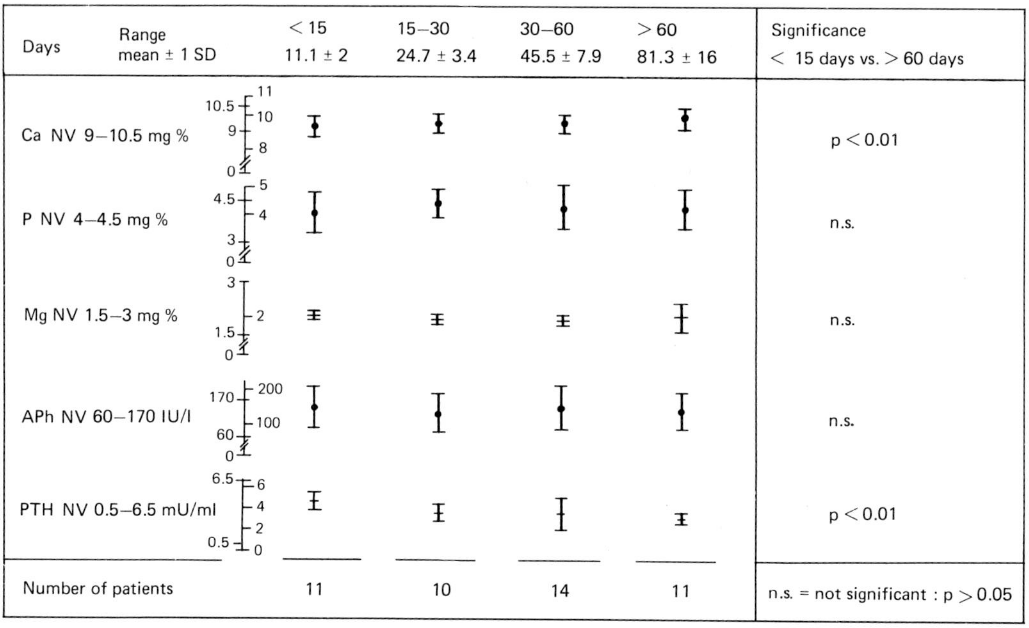

Fig. 1. Mean serum data of 27 immobilized patients divided into 4 groups according to the time of the first observation and to the period of immobilization. NV = Normal values.

Results and Discussion

Mean serum data at the time of the first observation in 27 patients immobilized for 32.7 ± 27.6 days (mean ± 1 SD) were normal as follows: Ca 9.49 ± 0.64mg%, P 4.2 ± 0.69, Mg 1.65 ± 0.14 mg%, APh 161 ± 60IU/l, PTH 3.9 ± 1mU/ml. Fasting U_{Ca}/U_{Cr} (0.194 ± 0.121) and U_{OHPr}/U_{Cr}, (0.053 ± 0.032) were increased. The renal phosphorus threshold (4.28 ± 1.06) reached the upper normal limits, while the MgEI (0.048 ± 0.016) was normal. These data show the occurrence of dismetabolisms although they mainly focus a static situation during a dynamic pathologic sequence. To study this sequence of events, patients were divided into 4 groups according to the time of the first observation and to the duration of immobilization. In all groups, mean serum values for Ca, P, Mg, APh and PTH were constantly normal (fig. 1). Of interest, serum Ca in patients immobilized for less than 15 days was reduced (9.25 ± 0.55mg%) as compared with patients with more than 60 days immobilization (10.06 ± 0.6mg%). In this latter group, PTH levels were

Table I. Mean excretion data of 27 immobilized patients divided into 4 groups according to the time of the first observation and to the period of immobilization

Days		U_{Ca}/U_{Cr} (n.v. < 0.150 mg %/mg %)	U_{OHPr}/U_{Cr} (n.v. < 0.03 mg %/mg %)	$TmPO_4/GFR$ (n.v. 2.5–4.2 mg/100 ml GF)	MgEl (0.025–0.1 mg/100 ml GF)	Number of patients
Range	<15	0.125 ± 0.08	0.043 ± 0.02	4.1 ± 1.1	0.042 ± 0.007	11
Mean ± 1 SD	11.1 ± 2					
Range	15–30	0.210 ± 0.11	0.055 ± 0.02	4.2 ± 0.7	0.052 ± 0.020	10
Mean ± 1 SD	24.7 ± 3.4					
Range	30–60	0.233 ± 0.13	0.056 ± 0.03	4.4 ± 1.2	0.037 ± 0.010	14
Mean ± 1 SD	45.5 ± 7.9					
Range	>60	0.242 ± 0.09	0.060 ± 0.03	4.5 ± 1.1	0.053 ± 0.016	11
Mean ± 1 SD	81.3 ± 16					

lower (3.2 ± 0.59 mU/ml) than in the former patients (4.72 ± 0.71 mU/ml). In patients with less than 15 days immobilization, U_{Ca}/U_{Cr} was normal, whereas U_{OHPr}/U_{Cr} was increased (table I). However, in the case of more prolonged immobilization, also U_{Ca}/U_{Cr} as well as U_{OHPr} became pathologic. Renal phosphorus threshold tended to progressively increase beyond the upper normal limits. MgEI was constantly normal. No statistically significant variation in U_{Ca}/U_{Cr}, U_{OHPr}/U_{Cr} were detected in regard to sex and age. On the whole, these data are in agreement with the histologic observations by *Minaire* et al. [1], whose studies on immobilized patients showed an altered bone turnover that was related to increased bone resorption and reduced bone synthesis. The comparison of U_{Ca}/U_{Cr} with U_{OHPr}/U_{Cr} showed that bone alterations were not only early events but that a pathophysiologic sequence may be envisaged. Hypercalciuria follows increased bone resorption. Increased urinary Ca excretion may be of the resorptive type. Contrary to the hypercalciuria classically associated with hyperparathyroidism, immobilization-induced hypercalciuria is characterized by normal serum PTH levels that tend to progressively decrease and by increased renal phosphorus threshold (fig. 1; table I).

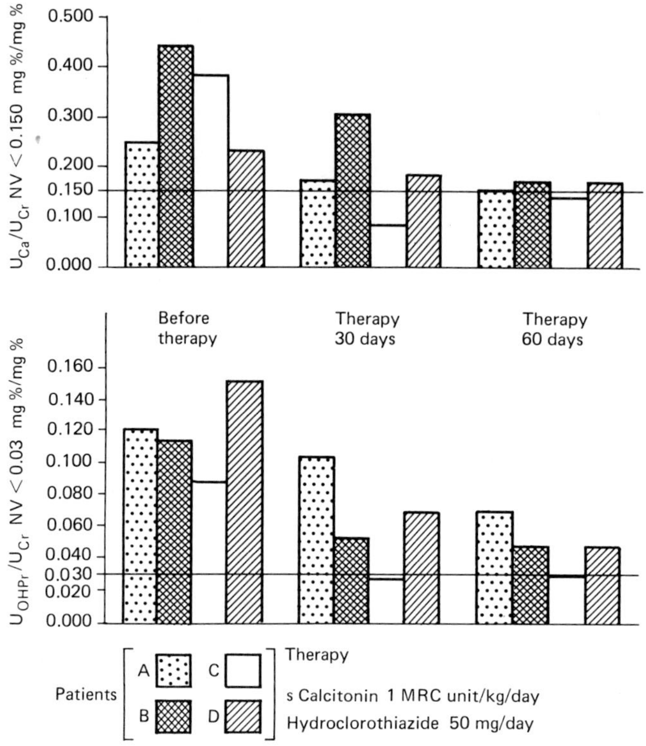

Fig. 2. Results obtained after treatment with synthetic salmon calcitonin and hydrochlorothiazide in 4 patients immobilized for different periods of time. NV = Normal values.

Conclusions

These results stimulated us to start calcitonin and thiazides in immobilized patients on the basis of its inhibition of bone resorption and of their hypocalciuric effect, respectively. The aim of these studies was to adopt a specific treatment of bone pathology and of urolithiasis prevention. Based on these theoretical considerations, synthetic salmon calcitonin and hydrochlorothiazide were given to 4 patients (2 M, 2 F, age range: 20–60 years; immobilized for 24–99 days before starting this therapy). For all these patients, a prolonged period of immobilization could be foreseen. Salmon calcitonin (1 MRC unit/kg/day) associated with hydrochlorothiazide (50 mg/day brought, in 1 month, the studied parameters back to normal values in 1 patient. In the other 3, amelioration of these parameters became evident 1 month after beginning therapy. The signs of amelioration were further consolidated after 2 months of therapy (fig. 2). On the whole, these results show the possibility to keep under control the metabolic abnormalities induced by immobilization and suggest a preventive treatment. However, these are preliminary data that need further confirmation.

References

1 Minaire, P.; Meunière, P.; Eduard, C.; Bernard, J.; Curprone, P.; Bourret, J.: Quantitative histological data on disuse osteoporosis. Comparison with biological data. Calcif. Tissue Res. *17*: 57–73 (1974).

2 Nordin, B.E.C.; Horsman, A.; Aaron, J.: Diagnostic procedures; in Nordin, Calcium, phosphate and magnesium metabolism, pp. 469–524 (Churchill Livingstone, Edinburgh 1976).

3 Stewart, A.F.; Adler, M.; Byers, C.M.; Segre, G.V.; Broadlis, A.: Calcium homeostasis in immobilization. An example of resorptive hypercalciuria. New Engl. J. Med. *19*: 1136–1140 (1982).

4 Walton, R.J.; Bijovet, O.L.M.: Nomogram for derivation of renal threshold phosphate concentration. Lancet *ii*: 309–310 (1975).

Alberto Jeantet, MD, Cattedra di Nefrologia, Divisione di Nefrologia e Dialisi, Ospedale Maggiore Molinette, Corso Polonia 14, I-10126 Torino (Italy)

Contr. Nephrol., vol. 37, pp. 36–40 (Karger, Basel 1984)

Hourly Urate Excretion in Patients with Calcium Oxalate Stone Disease[1]

Hans-Göran Tiselius[a], *Lasse Larsson*[b]

Departments of [a]Urology and [b]Clinical Chemistry, University Hospital, Linköping, Sweden

Several authors have proposed that urate might be an important risk factor for the formation of calcium oxalate concrements [1–4]. Unfortunately a satisfactory mechanism for urate in this respect has not been presented, but different hypotheses have been put forward. Development of calcium oxalate concrements might thus occur by a heterogenous crystallization on nuclei of sodium urate or uric acid [5–7]. By binding of crystallization inhibitors to sodium urate, uric acid or possibly colloidal urate [8–11], a reduced inhibiting activity might increase the rate of calcium oxalate crystal growth. In several clinical studies allopurinol appeared to decrease the recurrence rate of calcium oxalate stones, especially when hyperuricosuria was present [12–16]. However, in some studies an effect on stone formation was reported even with a normal urate excretion [12, 14, 15].

The present study was undertaken in order to obtain information on urate excretion in calcium oxalate stone formers during the day and to define risk periods for sodium urate and uric acid crystallization. For this reason urine samples were collected hourly between 06.00 and 23.00 h and in one fraction during the night.

The pK_s used in the calculations was 5.47 [17, 18]. The solubility products for uric acid and sodium urate were 2×10^{-9} and 4.8×10^{-5} M^2, and the formation products 5×10^{-9} and approximately 130×10^{-5} M^2 respectively [18]. Figure 1 demonstrates the mean urate concentration in 31 calcium oxalate stone formers. The highest urate concentrations were ob-

[1] This study was supported by grants from Östergötlands Läns Landsting and the Wellcome Foundation Ltd.

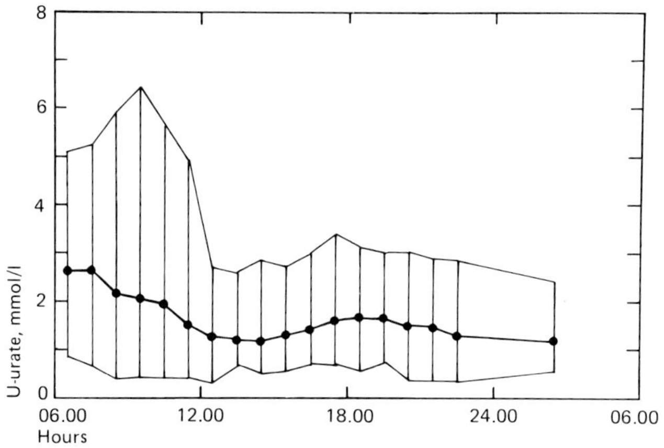

Fig. 1. Mean urate concentration (●) and ranges in 31 patients with calcium oxalate stone disease.

served before noon, particularly during the first 2h of the investigation, i.e. 06.00–08.00h. A high morning urate concentration was regularly recorded both in stone formers and normal subjects. Despite meal-related peaks of urate excretion, the urate concentration appeared to be inversely related to the urine flow.

One of the most important determinants of urate solubility is the pH. When the pH was measured throughout the day in freshly voided urine from 11 patients with calcium oxalate stone disease, the lowest pH level was recorded during the morning hours. The ion activity product of sodium urate (AP_{NaUr}) was calculated from the highest urate concentration, the highest pH, and a sodium concentration of 100mmol/l. The highest supersaturation and risk of forming sodium urate crystals appeared to occur before noon, but evidently there was also a risk period in the afternoon. However, the solubility of sodium urate at physiological pH is considerable and the formation product has a high value (fig. 2). When AP_{NaUr} was calculated by means of the highest urate concentrations, and the highest pH recorded at each hour, and with a sodium excretion as determined in one patient, a similar pattern was obtained. The level was clearly above the solubility product, but far below the formation product.

The lower the pH, the higher is the risk of uric acid crystallization. When the urate concentrations corresponding to the solubility and formation products of uric acid at mean pH were determined, it was evident that the most pronounced risk of uric acid crystallization occurred in the early morning hours. This was further emphasized when 51 urine samples col-

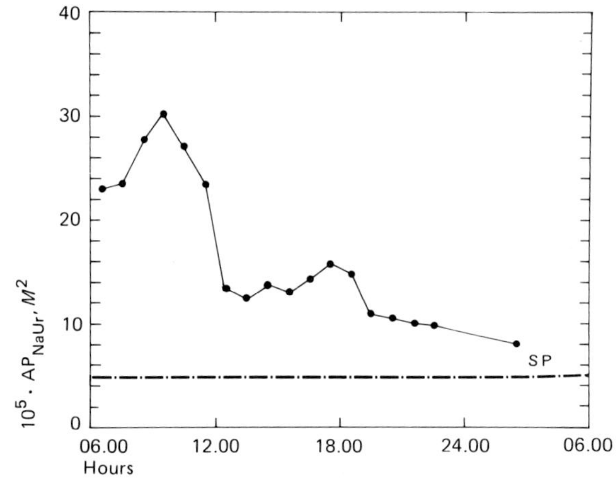

Fig. 2. Ion activity product of sodium urate calculated from the highest urate concentration, the highest pH and a sodium concentration of 100 mmol/l. The solubility product (SP) is indicated.

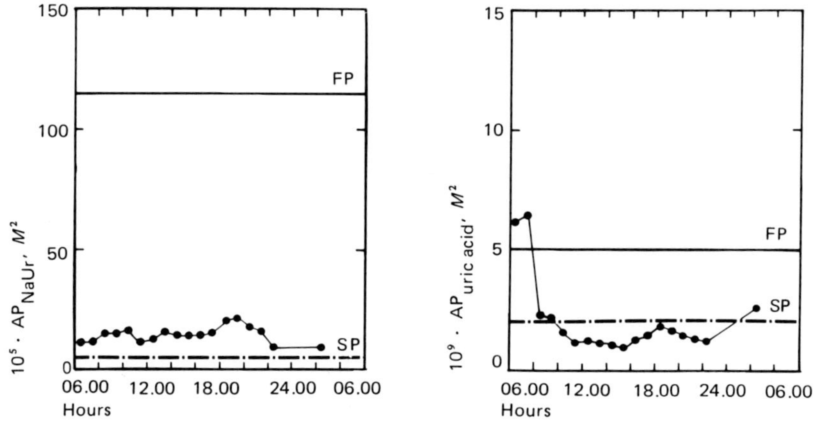

Fig. 3. Ion activity products of sodium urate (left) and uric acid (right) calculated from the mean urate excretion, the mean pH, a sodium concentration of 200 mmol/l at a 24 h urine volume of 1,500 ml. The solubility product (SP) and formation product (FP) are indicated.

lected from stone formers between 06.00 and 07.00 h and between 07.00 and 08.00 h were analyzed. At a pH of 5.0, 33 and 30 samples respectively had an ion-activity product of uric acid exceeding the formation product. The risk of sodium urate or uric acid crystallization is shown in figure 3. The ion acitivity products were here calculated from the recorded mean urate excretion, the mean pH, and a sodium concentration of 200 mmol/l at a 24 h urine volume of 1,500 ml. Apparently the risk of forming uric acid crystals is more pronounced than that of forming crystals of sodium urate.

The results in this study indicate that even with a fairly normal 24-hour urate excretion, there might be a risk of forming uric acid crystals, at least temporarily. Further studies are essential in order to demonstrate the frequency of uric acid crystalluria and whether this finding has any significance for calcium oxalate crystallization.

References

1 Coe, F.L.; Kavalach, A.G.: Hypercalciuria and hyperuricosuria in patients with calcium nephrolithiasis. New Engl. J. Med. *291*: 1344–1350 (1974).

2 Robertson, W.G.; Peacock, M.; Heyburn, P.J.; Marshall, D.H.; Clark, P.B.: Risk factors in calcium stone disease of the urinary tract. Br. J. Urol. *50*: 449–454 (1978).

3 Coe, F.L.: Hyperuricosuric calcium oxalate nephrolithiasis; in Brenner, Stein, Nephrolithiasis, pp. 116–135 (Churchill Livingstone, Edinburgh 1980).

4 Pak, C.Y.C.; Holt, K.; Britton, F.; Peterson, R.; Crowther, C.; Ward, D.: Assessment of pathogenetic roles of uric acid, monopotassium urate, monoammonium urate and monosodium urate in hyperuricosuric calcium oxalate nephrolithiasis. Mineral Electrolyte Metab. *4*: 130–136 (1980).

5 Pak, C.Y.C.; Arnold, L.H.: Heterogenous nucleation of calcium oxalate by seeds of monosodium urate. Proc. Soc. exp. Biol. Med. *149*: 930 (1975).

6 Koutsoukos, P.G.; Lam-Erwin, C.Y.C.; Nancollas, G.H.: Epitaxial considerations in urinary stone formation. I. The urate-oxalate-phosphate system. Investve Urol. *18*: 178 (1980).

7 Meyer, J.L.; Bergert, J.H.; Smith, L.H.: The epitaxially induced crystal growth of calcium oxalate by crystalline uric acid. Investve Urol. *14*: 115–119 (1976).

8 Robertson, W.G.; Kowles, F.; Peacock, M.: Urinary acid mucopolysaccharide inhibitors of calcium oxalate crystallization; in Fleisch, Robertson, Smith, Vahlensieck, Urolithiasis research, pp. 331–334 (Plenum Press, New York 1976).

9 Finlayson, B.; Du Bois, L.: Adsorption of heparin on sodium acid urate. Clinica chim. Acta *84*: 203–206 (1978).

10 Tiselius, H.-G.: Inhibition of calcium oxalate crystal growth in urine during treatment with allopurinol. Br. J. Urol. *52*: 189–192 (1980).

11 Fellström, B.: Urate metabolism and renal calcium stone disease. Scand. J. Urol. *62*: suppl. (1981).

12 Coe, F.L.: Treated and untreated recurrent calcium nephrolithiasis in patients with idiopathic hypercalciuria, hyperuricosuria or no metabolic disorder. Ann. intern. Med. *87*: 404–410 (1977).

13 Smith, M.J.V.: Placebo versus allopurinol for renal calculi. J. Urol. *117*: 690–692 (1977).

14 Brien, G.; Bick, C.: Allopurinol in the recurrence prevention of calcium oxalate lithiasis. Eur. Urol. *3*: 35–36 (1977).

15 Miano, L.; Petta, S.; Gallucci, M.: Allopurinol in the prevention of calcium oxalate renal stones. Eur. Urol. *5*: 229–232 (1979).

16 Berthoux, F.C.; Juge, J.; Genin, C.; Sabatier, J.C.; Assenat, H.: Double-blind trial of allopurinol as a preventive treatment in calcium urolithiasis. Mineral Electrolyte Metab. *2*: 207 (1979).

17 Finlayson, B.; Smith, A.: Stability of first dissociable proton of uric acid. J. chem. Engng Data *19*: 94 (1974).

18 Marshall, R.W.; Robertson, W.G.: Nomograms for the estimation of the saturation of urine with calcium oxalate, calcium phosphate, magnesium ammonium phosphate, uric acid, sodium acid urate, ammonium acid urate and cystine. Clinica chim. Acta *72*: 253–260 (1976).

H.-G. Tiselius, MD, Department of Urology, University Hospital,
S-58185 Linköping (Sweden)

Contr. Nephrol., vol. 37, pp. 41–44 (Karger, Basel 1984)

Urinary Calcium and Magnesium Variations during Sodium Cellulose Phosphate Treatment

A. Trinchieri, A. Mandressi, G. Zanetti, E. Patelli, G. Donghi, F. Rocco

Istituto di Urologia dell'Università di Milano, Italia

Introduction

Calcium and magnesium, the most abundant divalent cations in human beings, share some similarities in their metabolism. Moreover they are both involved in the formation of calcium-containing stones in the urinary tract. The urinary calcium concentration is an important determinant of crystalluria and renal stone formers have increased calcium excretion compared with matched controls [1]. On the other hand, magnesium is able to retard the precipitation and growth of calcium phosphate and calcium oxalate crystals under certain experimental conditions [2, 3], probably by forming more soluble salts with oxalate than calcium [4].

The reports published on urinary magnesium excretion of renal stone formers are conflicting: in some studies the urinary magnesium was reported to be lower, in other studies equal or higher compared with controls [5–7]. Indeed the urinary magnesium to calcium ratio is reduced in stone patients [5, 6, 8]. Zinc, a divalent cation present in small quantities in urine, was found to retard the precipitation of calcium crystals [9]: no variations in urinary zinc excretion are described, although the urinary zinc to calcium ratio in renal stone formers is reported to be lower than in controls [10].

In the present study magnesium, calcium and zinc excretions were determined after a short-term treatment with sodium cellulose phosphate (SCP) in order to evaluate the effect on stone prevention.

Material and Methods

20 absorptive hypercalciuric renal stone formers were studied (11 males and 9 females). Intestinal hyperabsorption of calcium was diagnosed with an oral calcium load test. All pa-

Table I. Urinary excretion of calcium, magnesium and zinc before and after SCP therapy

	CaE, mg/dl	MgE, mg/dl	ZnE, g/dl	MgE/CaE, mg/mg	ZnE/MgE, g/mg
Basal	0.170 ± 0.066	0.044 ± 0.022	0.49 ± 0.19	0.27 ± 0.07	3.20 ± 2.60
SCP treatment	0.083 ± 0.035 p < 0.001	0.014 ± 0.008 p < 0.001	0.40 ± 0.16 n.s.	0.17 ± 0.07 p < 0.05	6.80 ± 5.90 p < 0.02

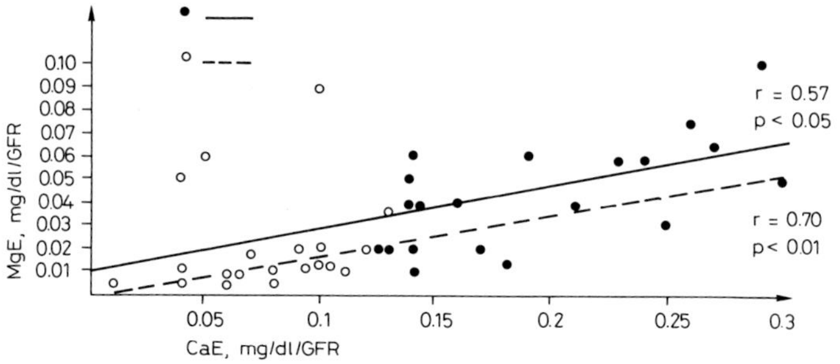

Fig. 1. Urinary magnesium excretion (MgE) as a function of urinary calcium excretion (CaE) before (solid circles) and after (open circles) SCP therapy.

tients were free of stones and urinary tract infections when studied. They were treated with SCP, 15 g orally administreted in three divided doses on free diet, for 7 days. Urinary calcium excretion (CaE mg/dl GFR), urinary magnesium excretion (MgE mg/dl GFR), urinary zinc excretion (ZnE mg/dl GFR), serum calcium (mg/dl), serum magnesium (mg/dl), serum zinc (mg/dl) were assessed before and after the experimental period. Zinc and magnesium concentrations were determined by atomic absorption, calcium concentrations by a Corning EEL model 940 calcimeter, creatinine concentrations by a colorimetric method.

Results

Table I summarizes the results. A statistically significant correlation was found between calcium and magnesium excretion on a free diet and a more significant correlation was found after SCP therapy (fig. 1).

Discussion

The present study, according to previous reports [11, 12], has shown that the short-term treatment with SCP markedly decreases urinary excretion of calcium. As recorded elsewhere, we observed no signs of enhanced parathyroid activity in absorptive hypercalciuric patients [13]. Sodium cellulose phosphate, an ion exchange substance, acts forming insoluble complexes with divalent ions in the gut, impairing their intestinal absorption and hence lowering their urine excretion. For stone prevention this mode of action might be beneficial by decreasing calcium excretion; on the other hand, it might be detrimental by reducing magnesium and zinc excretion.

In our study the reduction of urinary magnesium excretion after SCP was greater than that of calcium and as a consequence of this the urinary magnesium to calcium ratio was reduced. Since SCP has a quantitatively similar affinity for calcium and magnesium; we have to conclude that SCP divalent combining capacity reduces 'disposable' magnesium concentrations in the gut in a more unfavorable way than calcium, as regards their kinetics of luminal transport. Moreover, some investigators supported the theory that the calcium and magnesium intestinal transport systems are separate: in the jejunum a common saturable, facilitated diffusion mechanism dependent on vitamin D; in the ileum a magnesium prevailing transport system, probably independent of vitamin D [7]. Finally, magnesium and calcium share a common tubular reabsorption mechanism, but on very low magnesium and calcium diets, the magnesium balance is less negative than calcium, because urinary magnesium losses can be limited by a more potent renal mechanism [14].

The present data show, in agreement with the last observation, a positive correlation between calcium and magnesium urinary outputs and no significant fall in plasma magnesium after SCP treatment. Moreover, there was no significant change in urinary zinc excretion, so the zinc to calcium ratio is increased to a considerable degree because of decreasing urinary calcium. On this basis the long-term effects of SCP on stone disease are uncertain: a clinical trial demonstrated that in stone patients given SCP, without magnesium supplements, the recurrence rate was similar as regards the untreated controls [15]. In another study the reduction of stone recurrences was obtained with oral magnesium supplements and a careful choice of patients [12].

Conclusions

(1) SCP decreased urine calcium in absorptive hypercalciuric patients. (2) A greater fall occurred in magnesium excretion with a reduction of CaE/MgE. (3) Zinc excretion was unchanged, ZnE/CaE increased. (4) In ab-

sorptive hypercalciuric patients SCP may be a satisfactory form of treatment of recurrent stone formation if oral magnesium supplements are given.

References

1 Nordin, B.E.C.; Peacock, M.; Marshall, D.H.: Calcium excretion and hypercalciuria; in Vahlensieck, Urolithiasis research, pp. 101–115 (Plenum Press, New York 1976).

2 Bisaz, S.; Felix, R.; Neuman, W.F.; Fleisch, H.: Quantitative determination of inhibitors of calcium phosphate precipitation in whole urine. Mineral Electrolyte Metab. *1*: 74–83 (1978).

3 Meyer, J.L.; Smith, L.H.: Growth of calcium oxalate crystals. II. inhibition by natural urinary crystal growth inhibitors. Investve Urol. *13*: 36–39 (1975).

4 Desmars, J.F.; Tawashi, R.: Dissolution and growth of calcium oxalate monohydrate. I. Effect of magnesium and pH. Biochim. biophys. Acta *313*: 256–267 (1973).

5 Hodgkinson, A.: Relations between oxalic acid, calcium, magnesium and creatinine excretion in normal men and male patients with calcium oxalate kidney stones. Clin. Sci. mol. Med. *46*: 357–367 (1974).

6 Tiselius, H.G.; Almgard, L.E.; Larsson, L.; Sorbo, B.: A biochemical basis for grouping of patients with urolithiasis. Eur. Urol. *4*: 241–249 (1978).

7 Johansson, G.; Backman, U.; Danielson, B.G.; Ljunghall, S.; Wikstrom, B.: Magnesium metabolism in renal stone disease. Investve Urol. *18*: 93–97 (1980).

8 Oreopulos, D.G.; Soyannwo, M.A.O.; McGeown, M.G.: Magnesium/calcium ratio in urine of patients with renal stones. Lancet *ii*: 420–422 (1968).

9 Bird, E.D.; Thomas, W.C.: Effect of various metals on mineralisation in vitro. Proc. Soc. exp. Biol. Med. *112*: 640–643 (1963).

10 Surian, M.; Colussi, G.; Giachetti, M.; Masi, F.; Corradi, B.; Malberti, F.; Graziani, G.; Aroldi, A.; Minetti, L.: Urinary zinc and magnesium excretion in patients with idiopathic hypercalciuria. Effects of low-dose thiazide therapy. Mineral Metabol. Res. Italy *1*: 85–88 (1980).

11 Dent, C.E.; Harper, C.M.; Parfitt, A.M.: The effect of cellulose phosphate on calcium metabolism in patients with hypercalciuria. Clin. Sci. *27*: 417–425 (1964).

12 Pak, C.Y.C.: A cautious use of sodium cellulose phosphate in the management of calcium nephrolithiasis. Investve Urol. *19*: 187–190 (1981).

13 Mandressi, A.; Trinchieri, A.; Zanetti, G.; Aroldi, A.; Donghi, G.; Rocco, F.: Metabolic variations induced by short-term treatment with sodium cellulose phosphate. Mineral Metabol. Res. Italy (in press, 1983).

14 Massry, S.G.; Coburn, J.W.: The hormonal and non-hormonal control of renal excretion of calcium and magnesium. Nephron *10*: 66–70 (1973).

15 Backman, U.; Danielson, B.G.; Johansson, G.; Ljunghall, S.; Wikstrom, B.: Treatment of recurrent calcium stone formation with cellulose phosphate. J. Urol. *123*: 9–13 (1980).

Dr. A. Trinchieri, c/o Istituto di Urologia, Via Commenda 15, I-20123 Milano (Italy)

Round Table Discussion

Contr. Nephrol., vol. 37, pp. 45–51 (Karger, Basel 1984)

Early Dialysis

V. Bonomini, C. Feletti, M.P. Scolari, S. Stefoni

Institute of Nephrology, Dialysis and Transplantation, University of Bologna, Italy

We were the first to suggest early dialysis (ED) as the best method of artificial substitutive therapy in chronic uremia for preventing the appearance and the progression of most uremic problems [1–3]. There have been criticisms as well as appreciation of our first papers on ED. However, they concerned the idea of ED not our results, which unfortunately are still unique so that a useful exchange of information from different centers is at present impossible.

The criticisms raised by our first paper on ED [4–6] were partly justified and partly not as we subsequently made clear [7]. At all events the unquestionably violent reaction (the paper was called 'iconoclastic') [4] had the great merit of highlighting our contribution with its first-ever exposé of certain hard facts: (1) standard late dialysis (LD) fails to rehabilitate from uremia; (2) if started earlier, dialysis can prevent many uremic problems. Most problems that ED involves (ethical, logistic, clinical) have already been reported on in previous papers [8–11]. This report deals with the prophylactic properties of ED in dialysis itself and dialysis/transplantation integrated programmes.

Optimizing Technology and Optimizing Clinical Results

The fantastic improvement in artificial substitutive therapy in the last few years has been accompanied by no less fantastic improvements in patient survival. Though clinically rehabilitated, however, even to the point of resuming normal work, the survivors are by no means rehabilitated from uremia. Thus, dialysis technology brings about a double miracle: (1) *it keeps the patient alive*, and (2) *it keeps alive his uremia*. This is hardly surprising since uremia is due to the joint deficit of two renal functions (excretory and endocrine) and the so-called 'artificial kidney' can only offset the effects of the lost excretory function. If optimizing dialysis is to mean not only lengthening life or reinserting a patient into the environment of the family, but also guaranteeing full-time rehabilitation to society of a totally rehabilitated individual, we must admit we are doomed to failure from the outset. Even the most sophisticated technology in fact, will never reverse most uremic changes if they are already advanced once treatment begins.

Adequacy of Dialysis and Adequate Use of Dialysis

Two clinical and metabolic patterns tend to emerge in chronic dialysis, namely: (1) established and progressive uremia, and (2) 'prevented' and controlled uremia.

The first pattern is found with traditional LD (after years of LPD and initiated when the residual CCr is below 5 ml/min). In these patients not only do most clinical signs and metabolic problems present prior to RDT often persist on RDT; they frequently worsen as the years of dialysis go by. Intrinsic conditions of 'high risk' may be reached (progressive worsening in cardiovascular status, lipid abnormalities, osteodystrophy, etc.) both in dialysis itself and in dialysis/transplantation programmes.

The second smoother pattern is found in ED (begun at residual CCr of 10–15 ml/min; with little or no preliminary LPD; initiated primarily on the presence of clinical indications). The 3 main interrelated questions that have crystallized over the years are: (1) Is an ED approach ethically justified? (2) Economically viable? (3) Clinically rewarding? They have been recently reviewed and satisfactorily answered [9]. The prophylactic role of ED, however, needs further clarification in both qualitative and quantitative clinical terms. This is now possible in the light of the long-term results recorded in Bologna.

Issues Settled by Long-Term Study

Over the last 14 years we have put 82 cases on ED and 308 on standard LD. ED patients were: (a) those who complained of clinical signs of uremia despite CCr being relatively high (average 11 ml/min); (b) who had been on LPD for a short time or not at all, since they rebelled against dietary

Table I. Case material from the Institute of Nephrology and Dialysis, University of Bologna (1969–1982)

	Patients	12-year survival, %
ED	82	77
LD	308	51

Table II. Clinical 12-year results in a dialysis population

	ED	LD
Actuarial survival rate, %	77	51
Hospitalization time, days/year/patient	7	16
Full-time working, %	72	42

restrictions; (c) who voluntarily accepted ED after all pros and cons had been clearly explained to them. The dialysis schedule reported here was: 2 dialyses/week for 1–2 years and then 3 dialyses/week, or 3 dialyses/week from the outset according to individual needs. Table I reports the 12-year survival rate in ED and LD. Table II shows the differences in survival, hospitalization time due to clinical complications, and full working capacity. The hindsight of 12 years' experience affords the most realistic answer to the a priori criticism of the clinical role of ED. The results hitherto are clear: they indicate that ED is no longer merely an 'alleged' prophylactic approach, nor can it still be regarded as an 'experiment'.

Appropriate Comparison of Data

The clinical results (table I, II), though impressive, are open to the major criticism that they compare disparate case material. The key question is: what study model will ensure that retrospective comparative analysis of differing data in differing conditions has real statistical value? The biphase model we have already put forward [9] has been brought up to date for the purposes of the present study (fig. 1).

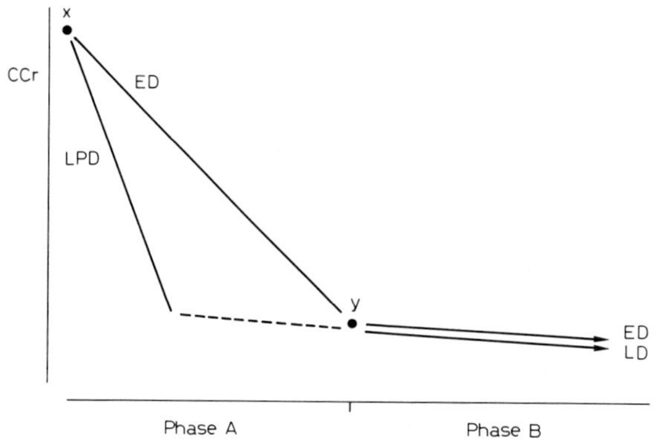

Fig. 1. The model employed in the longitudinal statistical comparison of cases presented.

Phase A compares ED (residual CCr 10–12) and conservative LPD patients (residual CCr 10–12) from that functional level down to the dialysis obligatory point (CCr less than 5 ml/min). *Phase B* compares the same patients thereafter both on dialysis and, in some cases, in subsequent renal transplantation. It is thus a longitudinal study on highly select material: the two groups in fact (deliberately restricted to 32 patients in ED and 57 in LD) met with the strictest criteria (homogeneity, comparability, length of follow-up) to ensure statistical reliability.

Phase A reveals a fact of undoubted pathophysiological interest in clear contrast with previous results [12]. Clinical data and residual CCr being equal, the deterioration rate of residual renal function is not accelerated by dialysis: the dialysis obligatory point is reached in 4 years by ED patients and in 1 year in the conservative LPD group [13]. Though repeated dialysis may indeed aggravate the reduction in residual renal function (especially when it induces marked postdialysis dehydration and, less frequently, hypotension), these clinical side effects need not occur if dialysis is performed properly and, above all, when massive ultrafiltration is not clinically necessary. This is frequently the case with ED, when, with residual CCr at 10–12 ml/min, diuresis is in general maintained, making heavy ultrafiltration unnecessary. Not dialysis, therefore, but technically incorrect or clinically inappropriate dialysis is to be considered a 'risk factor' for the deterioration rate of residual renal function in chronic renal failure. Possible responsible factors [13] for the 'maintenance' of residual CCr

Table III. Comparative longitudinal study of the same patients in phase A (residual CCr 10–5 ml/min) and in phase B (residual CCr 5–0 ml/min)

	Residual CCr 10–5 ml/min				Residual CCr 5–0 ml/min			
	ED (n = 32)	%	LPD (n = 57)	%	ED (n = 32)	%	LD (n = 57)	%
DBP > 90 mm Hg	6	18.7	28	49.1**	5	15.6	13	22.8
Abnormal lipid pattern	9	28.1	30	52.6***	10	31.2	33	57.8***
Impaired glucose TT	6	28.7	47	82.4*	7	21.8	28	49.1***
Peripheral vascular calcification	2	6.2	8	14.0	3	9.3	27	47.3*
Active resorption surface, %	4.0 ± 2.1		5.3 ± 2.7***		5.3 ± 3.8		6.8 ± 3.1**	
Hospitalization, days/year/patient	5.1 ± 1.3		18.5 ± 4.6*		4.7 ± 1.1		14.1 ± 3.8*	

*$p<0.001$; **$p<0.005$; ***$p<0.05$.

included an improvement in: (1) blood pressure control; (2) phosphorus balance, and (3) uric acid equilibrium. The extension of surviving renal function which ED entails, may also have wider clinical reflections. The renal activity prolonged is not only excretory but incretory. Since the majority of incretory renal functions are preserved at 10–12 residual CCr [11], and since the renal incretory products exert a number of effects on various biological systems, maintaining such levels of CCr for longer may mean greater peripheral alertness, sensitivity and response to metabolic stimulation.

Comparison of several clinical and metabolic parameters (table III) in phase A (dialysis nonobligatory) shows ED to exert the better control. The differences persist in phase B (table III) which compares similar dialysis patients, the only differences being *when* they started dialysis. These long-term studies on ED hence confirm previous results as to the lack of correlation with time between progressive deterioration of CCr and degree of many uremic problems [2, 3, 9]. The prophylactic action begins in phase A and persists through phase B (table III). If this is true, however, it is equally true that the inner mechanisms behind these ED properties are still a matter for speculation. Can the maintenance of residual CCr play any role in the prophylactic action of ED? It is hard to say with certainty. However, considering the wide spectrum of metabolic alterations in chronic uremia and in ED the better clinical and metabolic picture persisting even after the lower residual CCr has been reached (phase B), it seems likely that other factors are responsible. They may include: (1) the avoidance of the harmful effects of protracted uremia on LPD after the critical levels of residual CCr have been reached; (2) the better preserved renal and extrarenal hormonal equilibrium (erythropoietin, 1,25-DHCC, testosterone, PTH, gastrin, insulin); (3) the still connected reception and/or interpretation of peripheral messages suggested by the enhanced metabolic effects of supplementary therapy [9].

Whatever the exact mechanism may be, ED is invariably associated with an improvement in clinical and metabolic rehabilitation persisting both in dialysis and, in many cases, in subsequent transplantation. Some clinical and metabolic findings, in fact, differ significantly in transplantation from ED compared with LD, 2–4 years after surgery [9]. An improved patient rehabilitation follows, therefore, and dialysis re-entry, if needed, is made easier.

Conclusions

ED in the long-term confirms its validity in terms of prophylaxis: clinical uremia is 'prevented'; the progression with time is minimal. The prophylactic role is documentable in the years of dialysis and in many cases persists after transplantation. Since logistic difficulties may not allow a widespread use of ED, it should at least be adopted in: (a) young patients; (b) those with clinical signs of uremia despite CCr being 10–12 ml/min, and (c) candidates for renal transplantation. From infancy to maturity dialysis has revealed both clinical miracles and clinical limitations. The former are hard to explain. The latter not. But their very existence has brought about the idea of ED, which in our experience is the only way of matching technological optimization, clinical optimization, adequacy of dialysis and adequate use of dialysis. A priori denial of these assumptions without direct experience to back it up is, to say the least, scientifically unsound and ethically reprehensible.

References

1 Bonomini, V.; Scolari, M.P.; Albertazzi, A.; Bortolotti, G.C.: Basic distribution of uremic changes and their possible prevention by dialysis. Proc. EDTA *11*: 192–198 (1975).

2 Bonomini, V.; Albertazzi, A.; Vangelista, A.; Bortolotti, G.C.; Stefoni, S.; Scolari, M.P.: Residual renal function and effective rehabilitation in chronic dialysis. Nephron *16*: 89–99 (1976).

3 Bonomini, V.; Vangelista, A.; Stefoni, S.: Early dialysis in renal substitutive programs. Kidney int. *13*: S112–S116 (1978).

4 Berlyne, G.M.; Giovannetti, S.: When should entry into a regular hemodialysis programme occur? Nephron *16*: 81–82 (1976).

5 Maher, J.F.: When should maintenance dialysis be initiated? Nephron *16*: 83–88 (1976).

6 Scribner, B.: A critical comment. Nephron *16*: 100–102 (1976).

7 Bonomini, V.: Letter to the Editors. Nephron *17*: 235–236 (1976).

8 Bonomini, V.: Technology and the patient's management in a dialysis transplantation programme. Proc. 7th Int. Conf. on Recent Advances in Biomedical Engineering, Newcastle upon Tyne 1977, pp. 274–281.

9 Bonomini, V.; Baldrati, L.; Feletti, C.; Stefoni, S.; Vangelista, A.: Long-term early dialysis; in Giordano, Friedman, Uremia: pathobiology of patients treated for 10 years of more, pp. 133–137 (Wichtig, Milan 1981).

10 Bonomini, V.; Baldrati, L.; Stefoni, S.: Comparative cost/benefit analysis in early and late dialysis. Nephron *33*: 1–4 (1983).

11 Bonomini, V.; Orsoni, G.; Stefoni, S.; Vangelista, A.: Hormonal changes in uremia. Clin. Nephrol. *11*: 275–280 (1979).

12 Barsotti, G.; Guiducci, A.; Ciardella, F.; Giovannetti, S.: Effects on renal function of a low-nitrogen diet supplemented with essential aminoacids and ketoanalogues and of hemodialysis and free protein supply in patients with chronic renal failure. Nephron *27*: 113–117 (1981).

13 Bonomini, V.; Feletti, C.; Vangelista, A.: Progression rate of residual renal function in conservative treatment and early dialysis. Int. J. artif. Organs *5*: 93–96 (1982).

V. Bonomini, MD, Institute of Nephrology, Dialysis and Transplantation,
St. Orsola, University Hospital, I-40138 Bologna (Italy)

Contr. Nephrol., vol. 37, pp. 52–57 (Karger, Basel 1984)

Early Treatment of Renal Osteodystrophy

Otto Mehls, Eberhard Ritz

Department of Pediatrics and Internal Medicine, University of Heidelberg, FRG

The major problem in defining rational guidelines for early treatment of renal osteodystrophy is our ignorance with respect to the mechanisms which initiate disturbed calcium metabolism in the initial stage of renal insufficiency.

Abnormal Calcium Metabolism in Incipient Renal Failure

Elevated immunoreactive PTH levels are found even in early renal failure, i.e. patients with a GFR of no less than 80 ml/min [1]. Figure 1 shows our findings in uremic children. One might argue that such iPTH levels represent biologically inert material which accumulates because of delayed renal excretion and extraction of PTH fragments. However, in a previous study [2] we found woven osteoid and other evidence of excessive PTH action on bone tissue in patients with very early renal failure. Furthermore, *Kleerekoper* et al. [3] found increased nephrogenous cyclic AMP as evidence of excessive PTH action on target tissue in patients with a mean GFR of 60 ml/min.

The observation of early hyperparathyroidism in renal failure obviously raises the question of which signal triggers PTH oversecretion. Several authors [4] found low levels of both serum Ca and serum Pi in patients with early renal failure. This is also documented in figure 2. Hypocalcemia may represent a stimulus, perhaps not the only stimulus, for PTH oversecretion. Associated hypophosphatemia is presumably the result of the renal action of PTH [3]. Although fasting hypophosphatemia is uncontested, the argument has been raised that this may not be an adequate reflection of circadian serum Pi levels. We examined [5] the response of

1
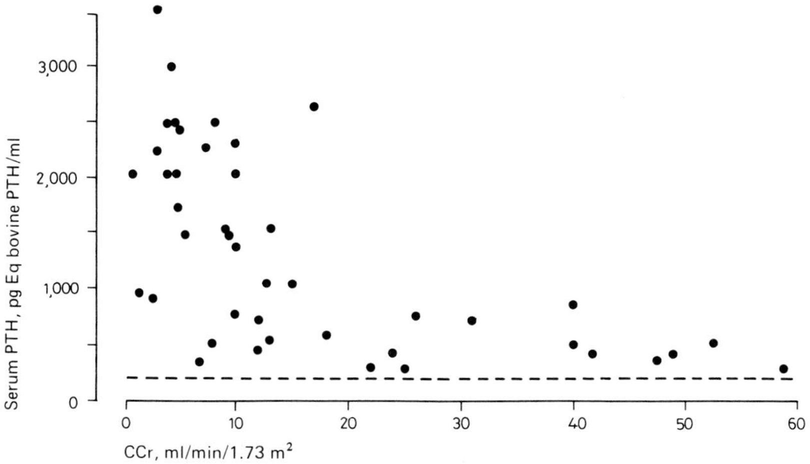

2
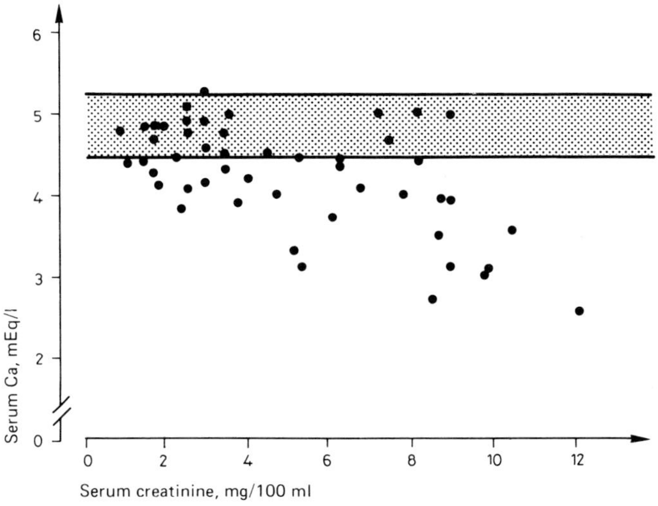

Fig. 1. Relation between endogenous creatinine clearance and serum iPTH (carboxyterminal assay) in uremic children.

Fig. 2. Relation between serum Ca and serum creatinine in uremic children.

serum Pi to an oral Pi load (fig. 3). Serum Pi was lower in 6 patients with a mean GFR of 70 ml/min, but the change of serum Pi in response to oral phosphate was identical with healthy controls. This finding is of note with respect to previous concepts of *Bricker* [6]. He proposed that with progressive renal failure adaptation of the kidney to increased Pi load is mediated

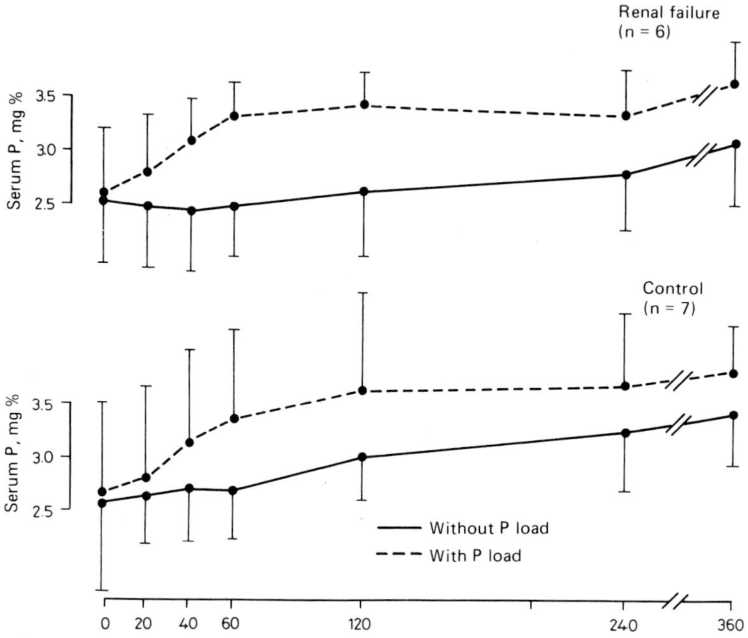

Fig. 3. Serum Pi with and without oral phosphate load in patients with incipient renal failure [5].

by PTH oversecretion. Although this mechanism is undoubtedly operative in terminal renal failure, as shown in experimental studies by *Slatopolsky* et al. [7], it is not demonstrable in early renal failure, presumably because the kidney adapts to changes of Pi load even in the absence of PTH as shown in the experimental study of *Carersazio* et al. [8a]. This does not necessarily imply that Pi has no role in the genesis of the early abnormalities of calcium metabolism, as discussed below.

Our observation of intestinal malabsorption of calcium in early renal failure [8b] suggested an abnormality of vitamin D metabolism. However, values for serum 1,25$(OH)_2D_3$ reported by *Slatopolsky* et al. [9] and *Ogura* et al. [10] were in the upper normal or normal range. This does not necessarily imply that 1,25$(OH)_2D_3$ does not play a role. Normal levels are certainly inadequate to the prevailing PTH excess, hypocalcemia, hypophosphatemia and intestinal malabsorption of calcium all of which should stimulate renal 1α-hydroxylase. It is of note that during repair of vitamin D deficiency, excessive levels of 1,25$(OH)_2D_3$ are present which self-correct hypocalcemia and hyperparathyroidism [11].

At present, we can only speculate as to the mechanism which prevents the kidneys to respond with adequate synthesis of 1,25$(OH)_2D_3$. *Llach* [pers. commun.] measured 1,25$(OH)_2D_3$ levels, iPTH levels and the calcemic action to PTH in patients with incipient renal failure prior to and after phosphate restriction. He found elevation of 1,25$(OH)_2D_3$ levels, decrease of iPTH and normalization of the calcemic response after Pi restriction, in agreement with the hypothesis previously proposed by *Massry* et al. [12]. These findings have recently been confirmed by *Portale* [18], but at our current state of knowledge it would be premature to advocate early phosphate restriction particularly given the hazards of phosphate depletion [13].

Prophylaxis in Incipient Renal Failure

It would seem rational, however, to correct early hypocalcemia and hyperparathyroidism by administration of 1,25$(OH)_2D_3$. Indeed, beneficial effects of long-term therapy were reported by *Healy* et al. [14]. Although it has been claimed that vitamin D (metabolites) are injurious to the kidney independent of hypercalcemia and hypercalciuria [15], this postulate is not supported by good clinical evidence and would be in contrast to previous pediatric experience with vitamin D therapy in vitamin D-resistant rickets. Such early prevention appears logical because normalization of serum calcium by prolonged vitamin D therapy in doses that normalize intestinal absorption of calcium [16] failed to simultaneously normalize bone histology of patients in late stages of renal failure. It must be admitted, however, that advocation of prophylactic administration of 1,25$(OH)_2D_3$, at the present stage, is a theoretical postulate which is not supported by controlled clinical evidence.

Prophylaxis in Advanced Renal Failure

In advanced renal failure, the tendency for hyperphosphatemia (fig. 4) makes the administration of intestinal Pi binders mandatory, since dietary Pi restriction is not feasible without the risk of malnutrition. As one single exception, use of dairy products may be restricted in uremic patients. The known hazards of aluminium intoxication resulting from intestinal phosphate binders [17] make this recommendation somewhat dangerous,

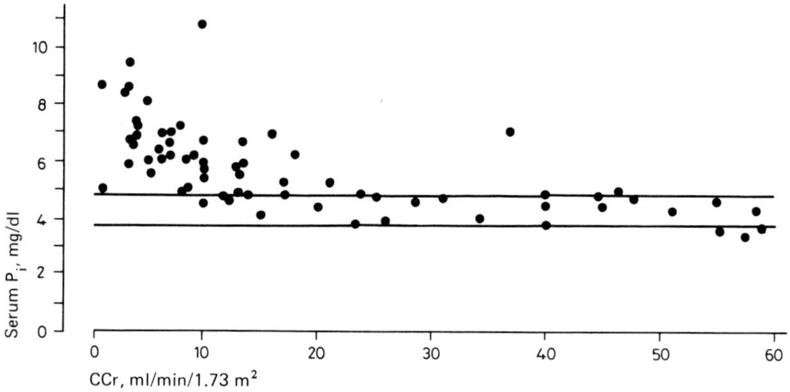

Fig. 4. Relation between endogenous creatinine clearance and serum Pi in uremic children.

but several non-Al-containing phosphate binders are available (calcium carbonate, magnesium-containing antacids) or tested in clinical trials [*Schneider*, pers. comm.].

Hypocalcemia, if present, should be corrected with calcium carbonate and the case for prophylactic $1,25(OH)_2D_3$ in this stage of renal failure is even stronger than in early renal failure. One should not forget the numerous causes of acquired vitamin D deficiency in uremic patients: administration of stimulants of the hepatic drug metabolizing system (phenobarbital), nephrotic syndrome with renal loss of protein bound vitamin D (metabolites), changed life-style with insufficient sun exposure, possibly diminished actinic generation of vitamin D because of cutaneous melanosis. In our experience, patients with analgesic nephropathy are singularly prone to vitamin D deficiency. Indeed, almost all cases with symptomatic uremic osteodystrophy prior to hemodialysis had been vitamin D-deficient patients with analgesic nephropathy. These patients, in addition, may also have an abnormality of vitamin D metabolism with lower $1,25(OH)_2D_3$ levels than predicted on the basis of GFR.

References

1 Reiss, E.; Canterbury, J.M.; Bercovitz, M.A.; Kaplan, E.L.: The role of phosphate on the secretion of parathyroid hormone in man. J. clin. Invest. *49*: 2146 (1970).

2 Malluche, H.H.; Ritz, E.; Lange, H.P.; Kutschera, J.; Hodgson, M.; Seiffert, U.; Schoeppe, W.: Bone histology in incipient and advanced renal failure. Kidney int. *9*: 355 (1976).

3 Kleerekoper, M.; Cruz, C.; Bernstein, R.S.; Levin, N.W.; Foreback, C.C.; Parfitt, A.M.: The phosphaturic action of PTH in the stady state in patients? Adv. exp. Med. Biol. *128*: 145 (1980).

4 Friis, T.; Hahnemann, S.; Weeke, E.: Serum calcium and serum phosphorous in uremia during administration of sodium phytate and aluminium hydroxide. Acta med. scand. *183*: 497 (1968).

5 Ritz, E.; Malluche, H.H.; Krempien, B.; Tschöpe, W.; Massry, S.G.: Pathogenesis of renal osteodystrophy: role of phosphate and skeletal resistance to PTH. Adv. exp. Med. Biol. *103*: 423 (1978).

6 Bricker, N.S.: An exposition of the 'trade off' hypothesis. New Engl. J. Med. *286*: 1093 (1972).

7 Slatopolsky, E.; Caglar, S.; Pennell, J.P.; Tagart, D.B.; Canterbury, J.; Bricker, N.S.: On the pathogenesis of hyperparathyroidism in chronic experimental renal insufficiency in the dog. J. clin. Invest. *50*: 492 (1971).

8a Caversazio, G.; Gloor, H.J.; Fleisch, H.; Bonjour, J.P.: Parathyroid hormone independent adaptation of renal tubular phosphate transport to renal mass reduction. Kidney int. *17*: 856 (1980).

8b Werner, E.; Malluche, H.H.; Ritz, E.: Intestinal absorption of calcium in incipient and advanced renal failure. Mineral Electrolyte Metab. *1*: 263 (1978).

9 Slatopolsky, E.; Gray, R.; Adams, N.D.; Lewis, J.; Hruska, K.; Martin, K.; Klahr, S.; de Luca, H.; Lemann, J.: Low serum levels of 1,25$(OH)_2D_3$ are not responsible for the development of secondary hyperparathyroidism in early renal failure. Kidney int. *14*: 177 (1978).

10 Ogura, Y.; Kawaguchi, Y.; Sakai, S.; Yamamoto, M.; Kimura, Y.; Oda, Y.; Imanura, N.; Tsukui, I.: Plasma levels of vitamin D metabolites in renal diseases. Contr. Nephrol., vol. 22, p. 18 (Karger, Basel 1980).

11 Stanbury, W.S.; Taylor, C.M.; Lumb, G.A.; Mawer, E.B.; Berry, J.; Hann, J.; Wallace, J.: Formation of vitamin D metabolites following correction of human vitamin D deficiency. Observations in patients with nutritional osteomalacia. Mineral Electrolyte Metab. *5*: 212 (1980).

12 Massry, S.G.; Ritz, E.; Verberckmoes, R.: Role of phosphate in the genesis of secondary hyperparathyroidism. Nephron *18*: 77 (1977).

13 Kreusser, W.; Ritz, E.; Boland, R.: Phosphate depletion, Klin. Wschr. *58*: 1–15 (1980).

14 Healy, M.D.; Malluche, H.H.; Goldstein, D.A.; Singer, F.R.; Massry, S.G.: Effects of long-term therapy with calciferol in patients with moderate renal failure. Archs intern Med. *140*: 1030 (1980).

15 Christiansen, C.; Rodbro, P.; Christensen, M.S.; Hartnack, B.: Is 1,25-dihydroxycholecalciferol harmful to renal function in patients with chronic renal failure? Clin. Endocrinol. *15*: 229 (1981).

16 Malluche, H.H.; Ritz, E.; Werner, E.; Meyer-Sabellek, W.: Long-term administration of vitamin D steroles in incipient and advanced renal failure – effect on bone histology. Clin. Nephrol. *10*: 218 (1978).

17 Drüeke, T.: Dialysis osteomalacia and aluminium intoxication. Nephron *26*: 207 (1980).

O. Mehls, MD, Department of Pediatrics and Internal Medicine,
University of Heidelberg, D-6900 Heidelberg (FRG)

Contr. Nephrol., vol. 37, pp. 58–61 (Karger, Basel 1984)

Prevention of Complications of Secondary Hyperparathyroidism in Long-Term Dialysis Patients

L. Bignardi, V. Cambi, F. Bono, F. Gardini, P. Zanelli

Cattedra di Nefrologia, Università di Parma, Italy

Secondary hyperparathyroidism (SH) in chronic renal failure and in long-term dialysis patients is often associated with severe bone and metabolic disorders. The purpose of this paper is to evaluate the rate and quality of PTH-dependent clinical problems in a controlled population and the preventive role of calcium and parathyroidectomy in reducing the most disabling complications.

Material and Methods

25 patients, mean age 44.6 ± 8.9 years, in chronic dialysis treatment for 10.48 ± 3.30 years, underwent parathyroidectomy (PTX). Dialyzer 1 m^2, Q_B 250, Q_D 500, time: 4 h thrice weekly; dialysate composition (in mEq/l): Na 140, K 1–3, Ca 4, Mg 1, Cl 106–108, acetate 40, glucose 1 g/l. Observation period before PTX 24 months, after PTX 20.3 ± 5.7.

During the years preceding PTX, therapy with vitamin D, calcium carbonate and $Al(OH_3)$ was recommended to all of them together with dietary phosphate restriction. The following parameters have been analyzed: serum Ca and P, alkaline phosphatases, PTH, body weight, hematocrit, mean blood pressure, urea and creatinine.

Results

The data given in table I were measured before and after PTX. Body weight, mean blood pressure, hematocrit, Ca and P, and alkaline phosphatases were statistically analyzed for a total period of 44 months (24 before and 20.3 after PTX); the results are described in table II. Only alkaline phosphatase showed a significant reduction after PTX. Phosphates were

Table I. Results measured before and after PTX

	PTH ng/ml	Creatinine mg %	Urea mg %
Pre	7.4 ± 2.7	14.0 ± 3.7	130 ± 110
Post	1.4 ± 1.1	13.7 ± 3.7	170 ± 130

reduced immediately after surgery, but returned to normal values with vitamin D therapy; hyperphosphatemia never occurred. The blood pressure improvement after PTX, as well as hematocrit increase, were not significant.

Discussion

According to present experience, SH proceeds through different stages: a first stage only characterized by increased PTH serum concentration, when GFR declines under 40ml/min [1]; a second stage when SH becomes symptomatic; finally in a more advanced stage, the insufficiently treated patient may present the most disabling consequences of the disease. Neither the diagnosis of primary renal disease nor the duration of renal failure appears helpful in predicting the severity of SH, when the patient first arrives at clinical observation.

Ionized calcium is the most important modulator of PTH secretion. However, in chronic renal failure, calcium intake should be particularly high because of reduced intestinal absorption [2]. On the other hand, the considerably high calcium concentration in the dialysate, i.e. 4mEq/l [3], was clearly associated with a good control of PTH production.

On the basis of these considerations a high calcium dialysate has been associated with 4h thrice weekly dialysis since 1971 [4]. Table III shows the frequency of signs and symptoms observed at the time of parathyroidectomy about 10 years after the beginning of chronic dialysis. The final indication for surgery was suggested by a clinically relevant combination of major and minor problems. Singly analyzed, most of the clinical signs presented a limited frequency up to 16%, while the operated patients were 14% of the total population. In order to evaluate the relationship between SH and uremic toxicity a statistical analysis on a long-term basis was planned: the operated patients have been followed for 2 years before and 2 years after surgery. The results, illustrated in Table II, point out that in a homogenous population, the importance of PTH as a uremic toxin seems

Table II. Statistical analysis, regression line and slope performed before and after PTX

		Body weight	Mean blood pressure	Ht	Ca	P	Alkaline phosphatase
Mean ± SD	pre	58.3 ± 7.2	107 ± 23	28.9 ± 7.1	10.6 ± 1.1	5.7 ± 1.4	247 ± 149
	post	58.2 ± 7.0	102 ± 12	29.4 ± 6.3	9.8 ± 1.2	5.3 ± 1.5	124 ± 81
	p	NS	NS	NS	NS	NS	<0.001
Regression	pre	y = 58.4 – 0.02 ×	y = 110 – 0.83 ×	y = 26.1 ± 0.48 ×	y = 10.4 ± 0.04 ×	y = 5.8 – 0.04 ×	y = 181 ± 16 ×
	p	NS	<0.05	<0.01	NS	NS	<0.001
	post	y = 58.0 + 0.05 ×	y = 102 + 0.06 ×	y = 30.4 – 0.22 ×	y = 10.0 – 0.05 ×	y = 4.7 ± 0.14 ×	y = 190 – 15 ×
	p	NS	NS	NS	NS	<0.01	<0.001
Slope	p	NS	<0.05	NS	NS	NS	<0.001

Table III. Frequency of signs and symptoms in 25 patients

	Cases	%
Major problems		
High alkaline pH	25	100
Bone pain	13	52
High serum Ca	9	32
High serum P	5	20
Minor problems		
Weight loss	4	16
Pruritus	3	12
Bone fractures	3	12
Metastatic calcification	3	12
Hypertension	2	8
Quadriceps tendon detachment	2	8
Blood transfusion need	2	8

to be overstimated. Furthermore, a stable body weight associated with stable predialysis serum urea and creatinine exclude any catabolic trends during the observation period.

In conclusion, SH in chronic dialysis patients up to 10 years is only exceptionally associated with the clinical picture of uremic toxicity. The most disabling complications described in the literature were rarely observed and always reversible. High calcium in the dialysate probably represented the most important support to vitamin D therapy in preventing the long-term complications of SH.

References

1 Arnaud, C.D.: Hyperparathyroidism and renal failure. Kidney int. *4*: 89–95 (1973).

2 Eastwood, J.B.; Bordier, P.J.; De Wardener, H.E.: Some biochemical, histological, radiological and clinical features of renal osteodystrophy. Kidney int. *4*: 128–140 (1973).

3 Goldsmith, R.S.; Johnson, W.J.: Role of phosphate depletion and high dialysate calcium in controlling dialytic renal osteodystrophy. Kidney int. *4*: 154–160 (1973).

4 Cambi, V.; Savazzi, G.; Arisi, L.; Bignardi, L.; Bruschi, G.; Rossi, E.; Migone, L.: Short dialysis schedules (SDS). Finally ready to become a routine? Proc. Eur. Dial. Transplant. Ass. *11*: 112–120 (1974).

Prof. V. Cambi, Cattedra di Nefrologia, Ospedale Maggiore, I-43100 Parma (Italy)

Contr. Nephrol., vol. 37, pp. 62–65 (Karger, Basel 1984)

Treatment of Renal Osteodystrophy in Advanced Renal Failure during Predialysis Time

Peter T. Fröhling, F. Kokot, K. Vetter, W.-D. Hohmann, G. Werner, I. Grossmann, R. Schmicker, Kristina Lindenau

Working Group 'Conservative Treatment', Society of Nephrology, GDR;
Department of Nephrology, Silesian School of Medicine, Katowice, Poland

Introduction

Hyperphosphataemia, hypocalcaemia, increased levels of parathyroid hormone (PTH) absolute or relative vitamin D deficiency and a relative deficiency of calcitonin play an important role in the genesis of renal osteodystrophy. The treatment with a pharmacological dosis of vitamin D in renal osteodystrophy has been assessed from different angles. But a marked decrease of inorganic phosphate has been observed after the administration of keto acids in a long-term observation period and this in spite of the reduced dosis of phosphate binders [3]. This study aims at investigating the biochemical and histological findings under long-term treatment with a pharmacological dosis of vitamin D_2 respectively vitamin D_2 and keto acids in the pre-dialysis stage.

Patients and Methods

50 patients with advanced renal failure (GFR lower than 15 ml/min) were treated with a low phosphorus-protein diet (protein intake 0.4 respectively 0.6 g/kg body weight/day) and a pharmacological dosis of vitamin D_2 for more than 12 months. The determination of the vitamin D_2 dosis was suited to individual demands and ranged from 20,000 to 120,000 U/day. 27 patients received a mixture of amino acids and keto acids as calcium salts, corresponding to 0.5 g N and 0.6 g calcium/day. 27 patients without vitamin D_2 treatment and without protein restriction served as control group. Transiliacal bone control biopsies were performed after 12 months on 39 patients who had been on vitamin D_2 treatment only, and on all patients who had had the combined treatment. PTH and calcitonin were investigated by radioimmunological analysis and 25-hydroxycholecalciferol was investigated by a radiocompetitive method. The bone mineral content (BMC) was measured by a photonic absorption method.

Table I. Histological findings

	n	Normal	Osteo-fibrosis	Osteo-idosis	Mixed form
Control group	27	0	3	1	23
Vitamin D only	50	9	1	23	17
Vitamin D + KA	27	11	0	9	7

Table II. Results of control biopsies after 12 months

	n		Normal	Osteo-fibrosis	Osteo-idosis	Mixed form
Vitamin D only	39	after 12 months	4	–	20	15
			6	–	15	18
Vitamin D + KA	27	after 12 months	4	–	9	14
			11	–	9	7

		Histological findings		
		improved	unchanged	deteriorated
Vitamin D only	39	8	27	4
Vitamin D + KA	27	14	11	2

Results and Discussion

The histological findings of the three groups are given in table I. It can be seen that all patients without treatment show hyperparathyroid changes, in most cases combined with osteoidosis. Under vitamin D_2 treatment normal bone was found in 9 out of 50 cases and osteofibrotic changes had been prevented in more than 50%. A higher rate of normal bone was found under the combined treatment (11 out of 27 patients). The rate of osteitis fibrosa had also decreased (table II).

12 months later these results were confirmed by control biopsies. In several cases a deterioration of bone disease could not be prevented by vitamin D_2 alone. An improvement was achieved in some patients only. On

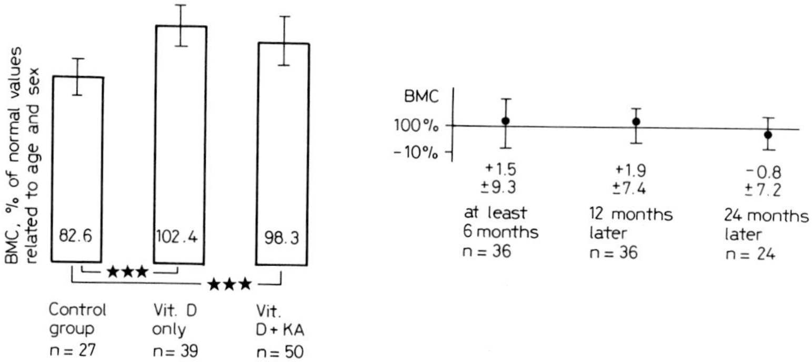

Fig. 1. BMC in patients with and without vitamin D respectively vitamin D and KA and the behaviour of BMC in the course of vitamin D treatment.

Table III. Biochemical data of investigated patient groups

	n	Creatinine mmol/l	Calcium mmol/l	Inorganic phosphate mmol/l	25–OH–D ng/ml	PTH ng/ml	CT pg/ml
Control group without vitamin D	27	937 ± 239	2.0 ± 0.5 ***	2.32 ± 0.58 ***	15.9 ± 10.2 ***	3.2 ± 1.2 ***	123 ± 69 ***
Vitamin D only	50	787 ± 274	2.5 ± 0.5	1.68 ± 0.42 **	82.2 ± 66.8	1.4 ± 0.9 **	580 ± 405
Vitamin D + KA	27	981 ± 354	2.5 ± 0.5	1.49 ± 0.32	51.3 ± 46.4	0.8 ± 0.6	584 ± 251

** $p < 0.05$; *** $p < 0.001$.

the other hand, the combined treatment led to a normalization of renal osteodystrophy in 11 out of 27 cases and a deterioration could be prevented in all patients except 2, in spite of the further decrease of the glomerular filtration rate in most patients.

Figure 1 shows mean values of the BMC under several kinds of treatment. Vitamin D_2 improves the BMC, and the values are stable in the normal range. There were no signs of KA influencing BMC (table III).

The untreated patients yield all the data typical of chronic renal insufficiency, i.e. hyperphosphataemia, hypocalcaemia, markedly increased PTH, slightly increased CT, and 25-OH-D in the lower normal range. Under vitamin D_2 treatment in combination with protein and phosphate restriction we observed a decrease of PTH and inorganic phosphate and a marked increase of 25-OH-D_3 and CT. Hypocalcaemia vanished. Moreover a further decrease of PTH and inorganic phosphate could be seen with the additional administration of keto acids. Our results show that the administration of a pharmacological dosis of vitamin D_2 leads to a normalization of calcium and a marked elevation of 25-OH-D_3 calcitonin. The constant BMC and the positive histological results compared with the results of untreated uremics indicate that this constellation has a therapeutic effect. The mineralization of bone can improve with increasing CT, which, in its turn, is due to the antagonism of PTH and CT. An effect of 25-OH-D_3 in the treatment of renal osteoidosis has been described by other authors too [1, 2]. Moreover, an increase of 24,25$(OH)_2$-D can be expected due to the elevated levels of 25-OH-D_3. Inorganic phosphate is influenced only by the phosphate restruction. This effect is insufficient and must be supported by the administration of phosphate binders in an adequate dosis (with the unclear risk of aluminium retention). Additional application of keto acids is followed by a further decrease of PTH and a decline of inorganic phosphate despite the reduced dosis of phosphate binders. The improvement of the histological findings is a strong argument for the introduction of the combined treatment of vitamin D and keto acids in the therapy of renal osteodystrophy in the predialysis period.

References

1 Eastwood, J.B.; Bord, J.: The effect of 25-OH-D_3 in the osteomalacia of chronic renal failure. Clin. Sci. *52*: 499–501 (1972).

2 Fournier, A.; Bordier, P.; Gueris, J.; Gebert, J.L.; Marie, P.; Ferriere, C.; Bedrossian, J.; De Luca, H.F.: Comparison of 1-hydroxycholecalciferol and 25-hydroxycholecalciferol in the treatment of renal osteodystrophy. Kidney int. *15*: 196–99 (1979).

3 Fröhling, P.T.; Schmicker, R.; Vetter, K.; Kaschube, I.; Götz, K.-H.; Jacopian, M.; Klinkmann, H.; Conservative treatment with keto acid and amino acid supplemented low-protein diets in chronic renal failure. Am. J. clin. Nutr. *33*: 1667–72 (1980).

Peter T. Fröhling, MD, St. Josefs-Hospital, Allee nach Sanssouci 7,
GDR-1500 Potsdam (GDR)

Contr. Nephrol., vol. 37, pp. 66–69 (Karger, Basel 1984)

How to Prevent Renal Osteodystrophy

Kristina Lindenau, F. Kokot, K. Vetter, W.-D. Hohmann, G. Werner, Rosemarie Buder, Inge Grossmann, P.T. Fröhling

Working Group 'Conservative Treatment', Society of Nephrology, Berlin, GDR, and Department of Nephrology, Silesian School of Medicine, Katowice, Poland

Introduction

Histological findings of renal osteodystrophy are present even in patients with only mild renal failure [4]. Increased levels of parathyroid hormone (PTH) were also noted in several patients with mild renal failure [4]. The starting point of disturbances of vitamin D metabolism in early stages of renal insufficiency was found controversial in literature [1]. Decreased bone mineral content (BMC) has been observed in patients in a moderate state of renal insufficiency [3]. Such data should lead to an attempt to prevent the increase of PTH and the disturbance in vitamin D metabolism as early as possible in patients with chronic renal insufficiency. The purpose of the present paper is to report the effects of therapy with early phosphate restriction, substitution of calcium and a pharmacological dosis of vitamin D_2 (ergocalciferol) on renal osteodystrophy in early stages of renal insufficiency. It will also describe the BMC, the biochemical and histological findings of patients treated with vitamin D_2 in comparison with an untreated control group.

Patients and Methods

The patients who were treated with vitamin D_2 were divided into two groups according to their glomerular filtration rate (GFR): between 42 and 24 ml/min and between 20 and 16 ml/min. The following parameters of bone metabolism were investigated: calcium, inorganic phosphate, alkaline phosphatase by standard methods, PTH and calcitonin by radioimmunological analysis and 25-hydroxyvitamin D by a radiocompetitive method. The BMC was measured by a photonic absorption method, and the bone histological investigation was car-

Table I. Biochemical characteristics in patients with mild and moderate renal insufficiency

	Mild renal insufficiency (serum creatinine <350 mmol/l)		Moderate renal insufficiency (serum creatinine >350 mmol/l)	
	without vitamin D	vitamin D treated	without vitamin D	vitamin D treated
25-OH-D, ng/ml	8.5 ± 5.6***	55.7 ± 30.6***	10.9 ± 8.1***	83.9 ± 55.5***
CT, pg/ml	296 ± 210***	635 ± 428***	282 ± 240**	530 ± 315**
PTH, ng/ml	0.62 ± 0.63**	0.25 ± 0.14**	0.98 ± 0.81*	0.61 ± 0.41*

*n.s.; **$p<0.01$; ***$p<0.001$.

ried out by transiliacal bone biopsy. The classification of the histological findings was performed according to *Delling* [2]. Type I fibroosteoclastic, type II osteomalacic, and type III mixed form of types I and II. The dosis of vitamin D_2 (Dekristol®) was given individually, while controlling serum calcium levels, and ranged between 20,000 and 90,000 U/day. The control group (without vitamin D) underwent the same diagnostic and therapeutic procedure.

Results and Discussion

Table I shows the biochemical characteristics of patients with mild and moderate renal insufficiency. It can be seen that the mild insufficiency group has significantly higher PTH levels and significantly lower calcitonin levels than the vitamin D-treated group. Under vitamin D_2 treatment the 25-hydroxyvitamin D_3 levels grew 6.5 times higher than in the untreated patients. In the group with moderate insufficiency there were significant differences between the calcitonin and 25-hydroxyvitamin D_3 levels with the same trend as in the mild insufficiency group. The serum levels of calcium and inorganic phosphate show no significant differences. Table II gives the histological findings of vitamin D_2-treated patients and the control group without vitamin D.

The results of the control group confirm the relatively high rate of renal osteodystrophy in the early and moderate stages of chronic renal failure. The consistent prophylaxis with phosphate restriction, calcium substitution and vitamin D_2 treatment in a pharmacological dosis resulted in a higher rate of normal bone. Rather unexpected was the decrease of bone mineral content in several patients with mild renal insufficiency.

Table II. Histological findings in the investigated patients

Serum cratinine mmol/l		n	Normal	Osteo-fibrosis	Osteo-idosis	Mixed form
<350	control group without vitamin D	53	5	12	12	24
	vitamin D treated	45	23	6	9	7
>350	control group without vitamin D	22	3	1	6	12
	vitamin D treated	49	4	0	34	11

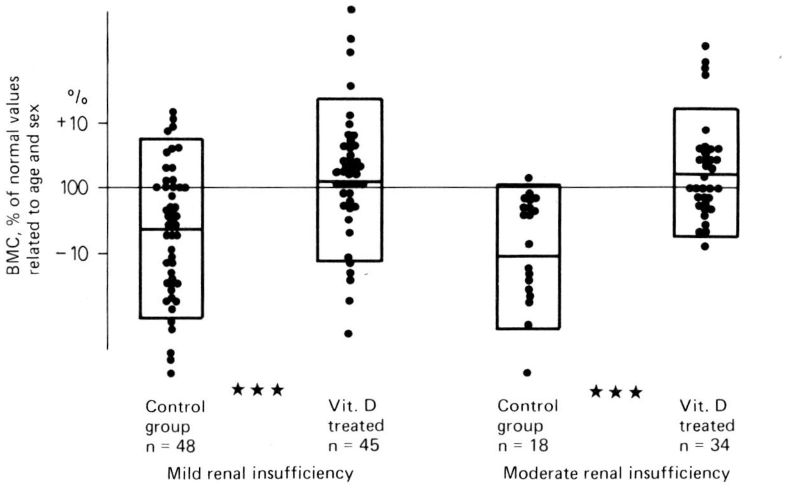

Fig. 1. Bone mineral content (BMC) of patients with mild (serum creatinine <350 mmol/l) or moderate (serum creatinine >350 mmol/l) renal insufficiency, with or without vitamin D treatment. $^{***}p<0.001$.

Decreased levels of 25-hydroxyvitamin D_3 and slightly increased PTH levels might be considered the cause of these findings in untreated patients (fig. 1). The advantages of vitamin D therapy in the early stages of renal insufficiency are the following: improvement of intestinal calcium resorption, increase of 25-hydroxyvitamin D_3 levels; suppression of PTH hypersecretion; elevation of calcitonin levels, and prevention of progressive bone demineralization. The necessity of this therapeutic strategy as a prophylaxis of renal osteodystrophy in the early stage of renal insufficiency can be recommended.

References

1 Avioli, L.V.: Controversies regarding uremia and acquired defects in vitamin D_3 metabolism. Kidney int. *13*: 8, pp. 36–38 (1978).

2 Delling, G.: Endokrine Osteopathie. Veröffentlichungen aus der Pathologie, p. 98 (Fischer, Stuttgart 1975).

3 Lindergard, B.: Changes in bone mineral content evaluated by photon absorptiometry before the start of active uremia treatment. Clin. Nephrol. *16*: 126–130 (1981).

4 Malluche, H.H.; Ritz, R.; Lange, H.P.; Kutschera, J.; Hodgson, M.; Seiffert, U.; Schoeppe, W.: Bone histology in incipient and advanced renal failure. Kidney int. *9*: 355–362 (1976).

Kristina Lindenau, MD, Humboldt-University Berlin, Clinic for Internal Medicine, Schumannstrasse 20/21, GDR-1040 Berlin (GDR)

Contr. Nephrol., vol. 37, pp. 70–77 (Karger, Basel 1984)

Definition of Biocompatibility

H. Klinkmann, H. Wolf, E. Schmitt

Department of Internal Medicine, Wilhelm Pieck University, Rostock, and Department of Medicine, Humboldt University, Berlin, GDR

In the last decade tremendous efforts were made in the development and improvement of life support systems and medical devices. One of the key issues in future artificial organ development will undoubtedly be the problem of biomaterial. The term 'biomaterial' is used for natural of synthetic materials that are used in contact with living tissue and/or biological fluids. In order to characterize biomaterials, the term 'biocompatibility' has been introduced as a quality concept. The term 'biocompatibility', however, has not been precisely defined and is usually considered to imply that the clinical use of such materials will not create effects which endanger the lives of patients.

From the simple clinical point of view, biocompatibility of a material requests the absence of thrombogenic, toxic, allergic, or inflammatory reaction, no destruction of formed elements, no changes in plasmaproteins and enzymes, no immunological reaction, no carcinogenic effect, and no deterioration of adjacent tissue.

Considering biocompatibility as the interrelationship between nonbiological surfaces and a living system, the following description of biocompatibility is possible. *Biocompatibility includes*: the energetics and kinetics of all physical, chemical, and biochemical processes at the interface between biomaterial and biological system during the time of contact and the direct reaction of the biological system induced by these processes at the interface; the sum of changes of physical and chemical properties of material, i.e., surface composition, surface free energy, corrosion, biodegradation, etc.; the sum of changes of the biological system outside the interface, triggered or induced by the interaction (toxic or immune reactions, cancer, etc.). To our knowledge the statement is justified, that there is no material available today that fulfills all the requirements stated above.

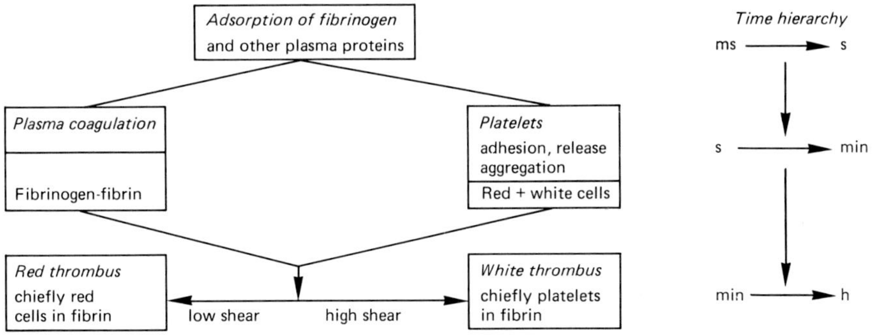

Fig. 1. Coagulation and thrombosis when flowing blood contacts synthetic surfaces. Modified from *Bruck* [2].

Progress in biomaterial research has mainly been hindered by the unavailability of internationally accepted methods for characterizing and testing of biocompatibility. Obviously the main problem in the determination of biocompatibility is the proof of unequivocal correlations between physical and chemical properties of materials and the complex reaction of the biological system during interaction.

From that point of view, biocompatibility can be characterized as an interfacial problem of high complexity. At this state of affairs these complex reactions are not understood in sufficient detail. Nevertheless there are some basic concepts which try to overcome the 'trial and error' principle in the search for biocompatible materials. Most ideas concern the blood-material interaction.

The initial events that occur if foreign surfaces come into contact with whole blood are shown in figure 1. This scheme was given by *Bruck* [2] and contains three major steps: (1) adsorption and subsequent changes of plasma proteins; (2) clotting of plasma proteins via a complex series of reactions involving the various clotting factors, and (3) activation of platelets and their aggregation with other formed blood elements. The formation of a red or white thrombus as a function of shear rate underlines the important role of hemorheological conditions in the entire process.

In addition to *Bruck*'s [2] scheme a time scale was introduced showing the time hierarchy of processes considered. The basic concepts for characterizing the hemocompatibility of biomaterials are based on the investigation of the interrelationship between these main events.

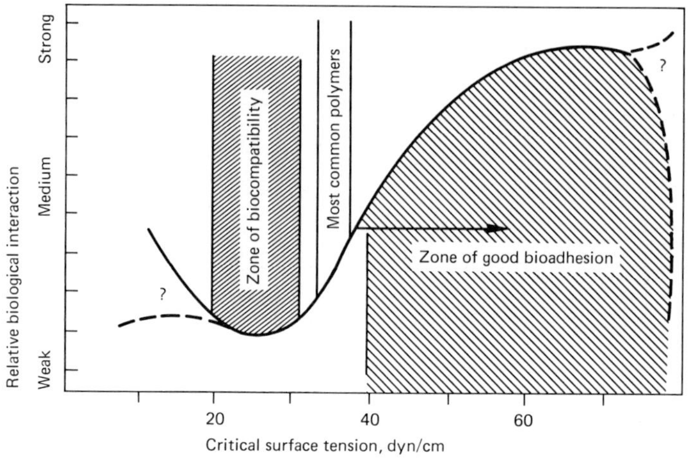

Fig. 2. Critical surface tension (dyn/cm). From *Bayer* [5].

Main Concepts of Hemocompatibility

Under constant rheological conditions, which cannot be considered here in detail, surface free energy, surface charge, surface roughness, and chemical surface composition are found to be the main factors influencing the subsequent steps during blood-material interaction.

With respect to surface charge as a parameter characterizing blood compatibility, the prevailing hypothesis for 2 decades has been that of *Sawyer* and co-workers [3, 4] which postulates: the higher the negative surface charge of a surface the better the antithrombogenic properties of this surface. Looking at this hypothesis in more detail it was found by several groups that the surface negativity alone cannot prevent plasma protein adsorption as well as cell adhesion, i.e., thrombus formation. One critical point in these studies, which are based on *Sawyer*'s hypothesis, is the fact that the surface charge density of materials and blood vessels was calculated on the basis of the classical colloid chemical equations, which cannot be used for biological objects because of the spatial distribution of fixed charges.

A second approach to correlate biocompatibility with physical and interfacial parameters was the observation that the clotting time of blood, platelet adhesion, and erythrocyte adhesion as well as the spreading behavior of other single cells seem to have an interrelationship to the surface free energy of solids.

From *Bayer* [5] a scheme was given that postulates a tentative correlation between critical surface tension of solids and their biological interactions (fig. 2). The region between 20 and 30 dyn/cm, where minimal cell spreading could be observed, was postulated as the zone of biocompatibility.

This concept was extended and accomplished by studies of *Kaelble, Moacanin* [6], and *Sharma* [7]. It was found that low dispersion-high polar surfaces provide surface energetics which appear to favor weak adsorption and retention of plasma proteins, i.e., a surface of poor hemocompatibility. Conversely, surfaces with high dispersion and low polar surface energy provide surface energetics to perform good blood compatibility. Table I shows some measuring values of surface energies given by *Sharma* [7]. The conditions postulated by *Sharma* [7] for good hemocompatibility are $\alpha_s \approx 4.7$ $(\text{dyne/cm})^{1/2}$ and $\beta_s \approx 3.0$ $(\text{dyne/cm})^{1/2}$ with $\beta_s/\alpha_s = 0.64$ approximately. According to *Andrade* et al. [8] materials will be highly thromboresistent, if they tend to have an interfacial energy of zero. The fact that materials with minimal interfacial energy like hydrogels do posses a low thrombogenicity supports this hypothesis.

Nevertheless, there are some limitations in these main concepts so far, which should not be neglected: (1) The surface energies are calculated from contact angle measurements which cannot be carried out under physiological conditions, i.e., in the presence of protein adsorption layers. (2) The calculation of surface free energies from contact angle measurement data is based on colloid chemical theories of restricted validity. (3) The term 'good hemocompatibility' used for the comparison with surface free energies of different materials is not quantified.

Unfortunately, from the in vitro or in vivo observations 'no or small platelet adhesion' or 'no or small thrombus formation' it cannot be directly concluded if the observed event (degree of platelet adhesion or thrombus formation) was mainly influenced by the hemorheological conditions, surface design, or the interrelationship between surface free energy of materials and formed blood components via the protein adsorption layer. The following examples illustrate the theoretical and practical problems:

In regard to the problem of changes in biocompatibility during an in vivo performance of a device, much attention has been given to membrane-filtering system such as dialyzers, hemofilters, and plasmafilters.

It has been demonstrated both experimentally and theoretically that, prior to the attachment of any cellular components, the surface exposed to blood first acquires a layer of sorbed plasma proteins. Even on the smooth-

Table I. Surface energy components for various polymers (from *Sharma* [7])

Polymer	$\gamma_s^d \pm 2.5$ dyn/cm	$\gamma_s^p \pm 1.0$ dyn/cm	$\gamma_c \pm 3.0$ dyn/cm	β_s/α_s
Silastic	19.4	9.0	25.5	0.68
Polyethylene	26.5	4.0	33.0	0.39
Polypropylene	26.0	3.0	30.0	0.34
Biomer	23.0	10.3	25.0	0.67
Avcothane	17.6	6.8	20.5	0.62

Table II. Fibrinogen adsorption for the Y56 resin coated with albumin (HSA)

	Adsorption rate based on	
Adsorbent	outer surface area, μg/cm²	dry wt., μg/g
Y56	3.51	491.6
Y56−1% HSA	0.74	103.6
Y56−5% HSA	1.03	144.3

n = 3.

est hemocompatible surfaces that remain free of adherent thrombi over a long period of time, this 'conditioning' layer of sorbed plasma proteins builds up and passivates the effect of the original surface. Thus, the state of sorbed protein molecules constituting the 'conditioning' layer is not only an important factor for the in vivo biocompatibility but also influences considerably the performance data of the device.

We all known the practical importance of this layer, often called the 'secondary membrane', for the efficacy of our membrane- or adsorbent-based detoxification devices. The relation between the biocompatibility and efficacy of a device as demonstrated by the membrane-systems will be another future key problem in biomaterial research.

Our group considers the rate of sorbed proteins as a reliable assessment of biocompatibility for detoxification devices. Together with Strathclyde University, Glasgow, we developed a simple miniaturized test circuit which permits us to assess the platelet and leukocyte fall in relation

Table III. Influence of albumin (HSA) coating on the in vitro fall in the level of platelets and leucocytes caused by hemoperfusion over uncoated and coated Y56

Adsorbent	Platelet fall, %	Leukocyte fall, %
Y56 uncoated	57.7 ± 16.3	59.3 ± 11.0
Y56−0.03% HSA	47.7 ± 10.4	50.1 ± 13.6
Y56−0.1% HSA	48.7 ± 16.4	56.9 ± 12.2
Y56−1.0% HSA	30.6 ± 19.1	59.1 ± 8.1
Y56−5.0% HSA	26.9 ± 9.7	56.7 ± 11.3
Y56−10.0% HSA	28.6 ± 12.3	57.2 ± 10.1
Empty columns[1]	1.8 ± 8.1	1.5 ± 11.0

Hemoperfusion time 120min, n = 6.
[1] n = 13.

Table IV. In vitro hemocompatibility tests

Platelet adhesion	+++
Activation of clotting factors	++
Platelet aggregation	+
Release of beta-thromboglobulin	+
Adsorption of fibrinogen/albumin	+
Resonance thrombography	+

High (+++), medium (++) and few (+) practical relevance.

to the absorption of protein, using ^{125}I-fibrinogen as a marker [for details, see ref. 9].

Tables II and III give the results obtained with different adsorbents. The results demonstrate that the adsorption rate of fibrinogen correlates with the decrease in platelet drop obtained with different adsorbents, thus proving that the rate of sorbed protein not only influences the efficacy of a device but also its biocompatibility.

Another example for the difficulty in judging biocompatibility tests for their clinical relevance [10] is the discussion about possible different biocompatibility of various dialysis membranes influencing the well-being of our patients. Leukocyte drop, neutropenia and complement activation are the reported results of the initial blood contact of cellophane mem-

Table V. In vivo hemocompatibility tests

Platelet adhesion (ex vivo)	+++
Vena cava test	+
Renal embolus test	+
AV-shunt obstruction time (ex vivo)	+
Fibronopeptide A generation	+
Dynamic tube test (ex vivo)	+

For explanation of symbols, see table IV.

branes. Pulmonary dysfunction, hypoxemia, urticaria, pruritus, wheezing have been claimed to be the result of impaired blood compatibility of cellophane. In some new membrane materials such as polyacrylonitrile and cellulose acetate these phenomena cannot be seen. For the clinician, the very difficult question arises whether these differences in certain parameters are of any clinical relevance. Table IV and table V try to summarize, based on the literature, the most commonly used test procedures. Our future efforts should primarily aim at the establishment of internationally accepted, standardized test procedures in order to make comparative studies possible. These studies should then be directed towards multiple facets of compatibility using whole native blood, because the preferred study of a single aspect of blood or tissue-surface interaction may often have been misleading as to overall compatibility.

References

1 Wolf, H.: Some basic aspects of biocompatibility (Auszug). Guest lecture, Int. ISAO Symp. Kinetic Modelling Artif. Organs, Rostock-Warnemünde 1982.

2 Bruck, S.D.: Current activities and future directions in biomaterials research. Ann. N.Y. Acad. Sci. *283*: 332–355 (1977).

3 Sawyer, P.N.: Bioelectric phenomena and intravascular thrombosis. Surgery, St. Louis *56*: 1020–1026 (1964).

4 Ramasamy, N.; Sawyer, P.N.: Interfacial reactions and thombosis. Bioelectrochemistry Bioenergetics *4*: 137–154 (1977).

5 Bayer, R.E.: The role of surface energy in thrombosis. Bull. N.Y. Acad. Med. *48*: 257–272 (1972).

6 Kaelble, D.H.; Moacanin, J.: A surface energy analysis of bioadhesion. Polymer *18*: 475–482 (1977).

7 Sharma, C.P.: Possible contributions of surface energy and interfacial parameters of synthetic polymers to blood compatibility. Biomaterials *2*: 57–59 (1981).

8 Andrade, J.A.; Lee, H.B.; John, M.S.; Kim, S.W.; Hibbs, J.B., Jr.: Water as a biomaterial. Trans. Am. Soc. artif. internal Organs *19*: 1 (1973).

9 Falkenhagen, D.; Esther, G.; Ahrenholz, P.; Holtz, M.; Schmitt, E.; Klinkmann, H.: Blood compatibility and efficiency of different hemoadsorbents, Proc. Eur. Soc. Artif. Organs *7* 137 (1980).

10 Lautier, A.; Bui-Mong-Hung; Pusineri, C.; Jarry, G.; Laurent, D.: Short-term in vivo testing of hemocompatible materials. Proc. 1st Int. Soc. Artif. Org. Tokyo. J. artif. Organs *2*: 71 (1978).

Prof. Dr. med. H. Klinkmann, Klinik für Innere Medizin, Universität Rostock,
DDR-2500 Rostock (GDR)

Contr. Nephrol., vol. 37, pp. 78–82 (Karger, Basel 1984)

Cellulose Acetate Hemodialysis Membranes Are Better Tolerated than Cuprophan

A Difference in Complement and Neutrophil Activation

Peter Ivanovich[a], Dennis E. Chenoweth[b], Reinhard Schmidt[a,c], Horst Klinkmann[c], Laurence A. Boxer[d], Harry S. Jacob[e], Dale E. Hammerschmidt[e]

[a]Northwestern University Medical School and the Lakeside VA Medical Center, Chicago, Ill., USA; [b]University of California at San Diego and San Diego VA Medical Center, San Diego, Calif., USA; [c]Universität Rostock, Rostock, DDR; [d]CS Mott Children's Hospital, University of Michigan, Ann Arbor, Mich., USA; [e]University of Minnesota, Minneapolis, Minn., USA

Introduction

Neutropenia regularly attends hemodialysis using dialyzers with cellophane membranes [1–3] and results from complement activation which occurs via the alternative pathway when plasma contacts the membrane of the dialyzer [2]. Coincident with the neutropenia, mild pulmonary dysfunction is seen [3]; while hypoxemia may be partially explained through gas exchange (and consequent hypoventilation) [4], changes also occur in closing volumes and CO diffusion [3] and a similar pattern of pulmonary dysfunction may be seen in other extracorporeal circumstances in which gas exchange does not occur [5]. The leukostasis and pulmonary dysfunction of early hemodialysis are usually asymptomatic, but may cause symptoms in an occasional patient with underlying cardiopulmonary disease [3, 6]. We believe that some of these symptoms may be the result of complement activation and resultant stimulation of granulocytes.

In early animal and clinical trials of dialyzers with cellulose acetate membranes we had the impression that they were better tolerated than cellulosic membrane dialyzers [7] and therefore specifically studied their clinical tolerance and their ability to activate complement and granulocytes in a prospective fashion.

Materials and Methods

Patients. 13 maintenance hemodialysis patients participated with informed consent in a blinded crossover study comparing dialyzers with Cuprophan (Travenol CF) or cellulose acetate (Cordis Dow CDAK-4000) membranes. Dialyzers of comparable surface area and configuration were used, and their identity was obscured with aluminium foil. Patients were asked to complete questionnaires at the end of dialysis treatments, concerning pruritus, fatigue and sense of well-being.

Clinical Blood Samples. During hemodialysis, EDTA-anticoagulated samples were obtained from each arm of the dialyzer circuit at various times. These were promptly centrifuged and the plasmas were retained frozen (−70 °C) until assay. Assays were performed on EDTA-anticoagulated plasmas which were shipped frozen to the laboratories at the Universities of Minnesota, San Diego and Indiana, respectively.

Complement Assays. CH_{50} was measured by standard techniques [8]. C3 conversion was detected immunoelectrophoretically as previously described [9]. Granulocyte aggregating activity was used as a bioassay of C5a as previously described [10] and was recorded as 'ZAP units' [11]. C3a and C5a were measured by a new radioimmunoassay, as described elsewhere in detail [12].

Evidence of Granulocyte Activation. Peripheral neutrophil counts were obtained by standard techniques during hemodialysis. As a reflection of granulocyte activation plasma lactoferrin was measured using a radioimmunoassay as described elsewhere [13].

In vitro Incubations. The in vitro potency of the two dialyzers to activate plasma complement was assayed in a manner analogous to earlier studies [2, 5]. 1 g of Cuprophan fibers was minced and was incubated aseptically with 20 ml minimally heparinized (1 U/ml) normal human plasma on a tipper for 0.5 h at 37 °C. These plasmas were then decanted and compared with parallel blank incubations and with incubations of similarly prepared cellulose acetate fibers for the following evidence of complement activation: decrement in CH_{50}, and C3 conversion and generation of granulocyte aggregating activity (vide supra).

Results

Patient Tolerance of Dialyzers. Well-being, pruritus and fatigue at the end of treatment were graded better during cellulose acetate hemodialysis than Cuprophan hemodialysis by the majority of patients during the blinded study ($p < 0.03$, U test). In 3 patients during 24 separate dialyses these differences were particularly dramatic, and the Cuprophan run had to be terminated. In 2 others chest pain, nausea and vomiting occurred during Cuprophan hemodialysis, but did not preclude completion of the runs.

Neutropenia. Postulating that less complement activation might underlie the clinical benefit seen with cellulose acetate dialyzers, we first looked to see whether neutropenia was less severe. Indeed, this was the case. In 25 patients undergoing hemodialysis with cellulose acetate devices, the white count fell an average of 22.4% (±4% SEM). In contrast, the same patients, when undergoing dialysis with Cuprophan devices, experienced a fall in white count of 61.7% (±2.9%; $p<0.01$).

Activation of Plasma Complement by Dialyzer Membranes in vitro. In results analogous to earlier studies, the incubation of Cuprophan membranes with plasma resulted in a significant fall in CH_{50} (22±6%) and the generation of substantial amounts of granulocyte aggregating activity (36.3±9.6 ZAP units). In contrast, plasma incubated with cellulose acetate fibers showed only a 6.5% decrement in CH_{50} and only 5.9 ZAP units of granulocyte aggregating activity. Concordantly, in each of 6 plasma donors studied, incubation with Cuprophan led to more extensive C3 conversion than parallel incubations with cellulose acetate.

Complement Activation during Dialysis. Estimation of C5a concentration in dialyzer arterial lines by granulocyte aggregometry showed convincing difference between the two dialyzers. We therefore assayed C3a and C5a by radioimmunoassay, a newer technique which provides greater sensitivity and objectivity; these samples were obtained from the venous lines. During hemodialysis, plasma C3a level rose from a mean 401 ng/ml (±63 ng/ml, normal <200 ng/ml) to a peak of 6,325 ng/ml (±1,103 ng/ml) in patients undergoing hemodialysis with Cuprophan devices. In patients using cellulose acetate devices, the baseline level was similar at 426 ng/ml (±43 ng/ml), but the mean peak was only 3,637 (±605 ng/ml $p<0.05$). The levels of immunoassayable C5a accumulating in the patients' circulation were unimpressive and not statistically different between the two dialyzers.

Lactoferrin Levels. Since lactoferrin is a granulocyte release product with a long enough half-life to be assayable as an index of granulocyte activation, we measured its level in plasmas of patients undergoing dialysis with the two devices. Concordant with the other results, we found that only 5 of 12 patients undergoing hemodialysis with cellulose acetate devices developed abnormal lactoferrin levels, in contrast to 12 of 13 patients being dialyzed with Cuprophan devices ($\chi^2=7.35$; 0.001 $p<0.01$).

Discussion

A possible role of the complement-stimulated granulocyte in a variety of disease states has been a source of a great deal of interest and some controversy in the past decade. While study of this has included many diseases, a major area of interest has continued to be extracorporeal circulation, in which many of the early data were generated [2, 3, 5, 14].

Studying hemodialysis patients in a blinded prospective fashion, we found that intradialytic symptoms were consistently and statistically significantly less severe when cellulose acetate hemodialyzers were used than when Cuprophan dialyzers were used. We found this to correlate with a lesser degree of neutropenia, a lesser potency of cellulose acetate to activate plasma complement in vitro, lower plasma levels during cellulose acetate hemodialysis of the complement-derived anaphylatoxin C3a and a lower level in those patients of the granulocyte release product lactoferrin. We conclude that the cellulose acetate device is in fact better tolerated in terms of patient symptoms than the Cuprophan device, and we postulate that this benefit likely derives from the now demonstrated lesser ability of the cellulose acetate device to activate complement and in turn to activate granulocytes.

Acknowledgements

The authors thank *Gordon Fleig* of Cordis Dow, *Hsin-Hsin Yung*, *Patricia Coppo*, MS, and *Nan Wilson*, MLA, who provided technical assistance. Dr. Hammerschmidt is the recipient of a Young Investigator Research Award from the National Institutes of Health (USA) and is further supported by NIH grants HL-26218 and HL-19725.

References

1 Kaplow, L.S.; Goffinet, J.A.: Profound neutropenia during the early phase of hemodialysis. J. Am. med. Ass. *203*: 1135–1137 (1968).

2 Craddock, P.R.; Fehr, J.; Dalmasso, A.P.; Brigham, K.L.; Jacob, H.S.: Hemodialysis leukopenia: pulmonary vascular leukostasis resulting from complement activation by dialyzer cellophane membranes. J. clin. Invest. *59*: 879–888 (1977).

3 Craddock, P.R.; Fehr, J.; Brigham, K.L.; Kroneberg, R.S.; Jacob, H.S.: Complement and leukocyte-mediated pulmonary dysfunction in hemodialysis. New Engl. J. Med. *296*: 769–774 (1977).

4 Dolan, M.J.; Whipp, B.J.; Davidson, W.D.; Weitzman, R.E.; Wasserman, K.: Hypopnea associated with acetate hemodialysis: carbon dioxide-flow-dependent ventilation. New Engl. J. Med. *305*: 72–75 (1981).

5 Hammerschmidt, D.E.; Craddock, P.R.; McCullough, J.J.; Kronenberg, R.S.; Dalmasso, A.P.; Jacob, H.S.: Complement activation and pulmonary leukostasis during nylon-fiber filtration leukapheresis. Blood *51*: 721–730 (1978).

6 Jacob, H.S.; Hammerschmidt, D.E.; Grouse, L.D.: Complement-induced granulocyte aggregation. Importance in myocardial infarction and shock lung (clinical perspectives). J. Am. med. Ass. *245*: 2013–2017 (1981).

7 Ivanovich, P.; Xu, C.G.; Kwaan, H.C.; Hathiwala, S.: Studies of coagulation and platelet functions in heparin-free hemodialysis. Nephron *33*: 116–120 (1983).

8 Nelson, R.A.; Jensen, J.; Gigli, I.; Tanura, N.: Methods for the separation, purification and measurement of the nine components of hemolytic complement in guinea pig serum. Immunochemistry *3*: 111–135 (1966).

9 Hammerschmidt, D.E.; Greenberg, C.S.; Yamada, O.; Craddock, P.R.; Jacob, H.S.: Cholesterol and atheroma lipids activate complement and stimulate granulocytes. J. Lab. clin. Med. *98*: 68–77 (1981).

10 Hammerschmidt, D.E.; Bowers, T.K.; Lammi-Keefe, C.J.; Jacob, H.S.; Craddock, P.R.: Granulocyte aggregometry: a sensitive technique for the detection of C5a and complement activation. Blood *55*: 898–902 (1980).

11 Hammerschmidt, D.E.; Weaver, L.J.; Hudson, L.D.; Craddock, P.R.; Jacob, H.S.: Association of complement activation and elevated plasma-C5a with adult respiratory distress syndome: pathophysiologic relevance and possible prognostic value. Lancet *i*: 947–949 (1980).

12 Hugli, T.E.; Chenoweth, D.E.: Biologically active peptides of complement: techniques and significance of C3a and C5a measurements; in Nakamura, Dito, Tucker, Immunoassays: clinical laboratory techniques for the 1980s, pp. 443–460 (Liss, New York 1980).

13 Oseas, R.; Yan, H.H.; Baehner, R.L.; Boxer, L.A.: Lactoferrin: a promotor of polymorphonuclear leukocyte adhesiveness. Blood *57*: 939–945 (1981).

14 Malchesky, P.S.; Asanuma, Y.; Nose, Y.; Hammerschmidt, D.E.: On-line filtration hemoperfusion with sorbent treatment of filtered plasma. Am. Soc. artif. int. Org. Trans. *26*: 541–545 (1980).

P. Ivanovich, MD, Chief, Hemodialysis Unit, Veterans Administration Lakeside Medical Center, The Medical School, 333 East Huron Street, Chicago, IL 60611 (USA)

Contr. Nephrol., vol. 37, pp. 83–88 (Karger, Basel 1984)

Neutrophil and Eosinophil Degranulation by Hemodialysis Membranes

Bo G. Danielson, Roger Hällgren, Per Venge

Department of Internal Medicine, University Hospital, Uppsala, Sweden

Profound but transient neutropenia during the early phase of hemodialysis has been observed for several years [1–4]. The disappearance of neutrophils seems to reflect a trapping of the cells in the lungs. Previous studies have implicated activated components of complement generated by exposure of plasma to the dialyzer membrane as responsible for this neutropenia. Such activated components produce increased adhesiveness of neutrophils making them more apt to fasten in the microvessels of the lungs. This is accompanied by pulmonary dysfunction and hypoxemia. The mechanisms are unknown but it is not unlikely that it is mediated by tissue-destructive substances released from triggered granulocytes. Local secretion by granulocytes in the lungs is anticipated to be reflected by increased circulating levels of granulocyte secretory products.

In order to investigate whether hemodialysis was accompanied by signs of neutrophil or eosinophil degranulation, the following experiments were performed. Intracellular contents and circulating levels of some granular proteins – lactoferrin, lysosyme and eosinophil cationic protein (ECP – during dialysis were analyzed [5, 6].

The primary role of polymorphonuclear neutrophils (PMN) is to remove invading exogenic organisms. They are a part of the defence system of the body against infection. The outstanding feature of PMN is their capacity to ingest and degrade microorganisms and other particles, the process called phagocytosis. The neutrophils also play a central role in the inflammatory process induced by antigen-antibody complexes. These complexes activate the complement system and also bind complement. Some of the activated complement components attract neutrophils to the site of inflammation. The attracted granulocytes ingest the deposited complexes and degrade them. When the phagocyte is overwhelmed by its phagocytic burden the granular constituents may be released extracellularly. Many of the discharged substances are proteolytic enzymes and are probably critical in the development of tissue destruction seen at the site of the inflammation. When activated the neutrophils secrete substances which are proteolytic enzymes. These enzymes are contained in two types of granula, namely the primary ones which contain different enzymes like myeloperoxidase (MPO), chymotrypsin-like cationic protein (CCP), collagenase and lysozyme, whereas the secondary specific granules contain lactoferrin and lysozyme.

In the first study 7 patients with chronic renal failure on hemodialysis 2–3 times weekly were investigated. Dialysis was performed for 5–6 h with disposable single-use dialyzers like Gambro-Lundia in 4 patients, Nephross in 1 patient and Asahi-filter in 2 patients. 4 adult patients undergoing routine peritoneal dialysis were also studied as controls.

The polymorphonuclear leucocyte counts, total mononuclear leucocyte counts and circulating levels of lactoferrin and lysozyme during hemodialysis were studied. Reduction of circulating PMN and eosinophils occurred during the first 10 min following the start of hemodialysis and was observed in all patients. After the initial decline the level returned to predialysis levels. The mononuclear leucocyte levels did not change very much. The pronounced increase of serum lactoferrin from the primary granules was observed 2 h from the start of dialysis. Lactoferrin remained elevated throughout the observation period. Serum lysozyme stayed within narrow limits and no significant changes were observed.

There was also a drop in the eosinophils. The ECP increased gradually during the first 2 h but declined at the end of the dialysis period back to predialysis levels. No apparent dialyzer-dependent differentes in results were observed.

In 4 of the patients studied the intracellular granulocyte content of ECP and lactoferrin was measured. Only slight and inconstant variations of these granular proteins were observed during hemodialysis compared to pre- and postdialysis values.

In one experiment fresh blood was circulated through the dialyzer without having a patient in the circuit. The serum levels of lactoferrin and ECP were measured 1, 2 and 3h from start of dialysis.

The serum levels of both proteins increased very much compared to the initial levels. Lactoferrin increased 14 and ECP 76 times and remained at the same level during the rest of the experiment. The lysozyme level increased by only 25 %. These results indicate that the neutrophils degranulate during the passage of the dialysis system.

In the group of patients on intermittent peritoneal dialysis no significant variations in circulating cell numbers or serum levels of lactoferrin, lysozyme or ECP were detected, indicating that dialysis itself did not result in a reduction of neutrophils.

Fresh normal human serum was complement activated by incubation with particulate protein A-IgG complexes at 37 °C. Addition to normal granulocytes of this serum resulted in granulocyte aggregation. Parallel to the aggregation an extracellular release of lactoferrin and lysozyme was noticed. The release of lactoferrin was about 30 % of the total granulocyte content of this protein, i.e. relatively more pronounced than the release of lysozyme which was about 10 % of the total intracellular lysozyme content. No significant release of ECP was observed. Lack of lactic dehydrogenase release ruled out nonspecific damage. Uremic sera, obtained prior to and 1, 2 and 4h after the start of dialysis, induced no granulocyte aggregation as compared to uncubated controls using non-activated normal serum.

From these experiments it could be concluded that hemodialysis gives a reduction of circulating neutrophils and eosinophils. With this transient neutropenia a significant increase in serum lactoferrin was observed, reaching a maximum 2h after the start of dialysis. At this time the increase in ECP had reached its maximum. The release of ECP started, however, earlier than the release of lactoferrin, indicating different secretion mechanisms. The lysozyme level did not change very much, probably as a result of the high baseline levels in uremic patients.

This difference could indicate different release mechanisms for these granular proteins. Recent data imply that activated complement components, especially generated C5a, induce the initial neutropenia during hemodialysis. Since complement-activated serum induced in vitro an immediate onset of neutrophil aggregation accompanied by cellular release of lactoferrin but not ECP, it is possible that during dialysis degranulation of at least neutrophils occurs in the circulation. However, one would then expect that the serum increase of lactoferrin would have occurred at the same time with the early fall of neutrophils, that is when granulocyte microaggregation may occur in the circulation. The inability of uremic sera, obtained at various times from the start of dialysis, to induce in vitro granular protein release from isolated normal granulocytes is a further argument against the idea that the granulocytes were degranulated in the circulation. The unaffected intracellular content of lactoferrin or ECP in granulocytes isolated from blood samples collected throughout the dialysis also suggested that circulating neutrophils and eosinophils had not been degranulated.

The inability of activated serum to induce in vitro degranulation of *eosinophils* suggests that these cells react differently than neutrophils to activated complement components. The absence of eosinophil degranulation in vitro is also strong evidence against the possibility that the observed increase in serum ECP during dialysis reflects an eosinophil degranulation in the circulation.

The degranulation of neutrophils and eosinophils during hemodialysis of uremic patients may occur in the circulation of the patients as a consequence of activated complement components generated by exposure of plasma to the dialysis membrane. Another alternative may be that the degranulation may reflect an effect of the dialysis membrane on the granulocytes. In order to study these alternatives we measured the intracellular contents and plasma levels of some of the granular proteins during experimentel hemodialysis without having a patient in the circuit.

Fresh heparinized blood was circulated for 2h through two kinds of dialyzers, namely a plate dialyzer with a cuprophane membrane and a capillary dialyzer with cellulose acetate as a membrane. Blood samples were drawn from the efferent blood line of the dialyzer immediately before and during the dialysis. Lactoferrin, lysozyme, ECP and MPO were measured by radioimmunoassays. There was no significant change in the neutrophil counts. The number of circulating eosinophils steadily decreased during dialysis and after 2h the count was reduced to 67% of the initial number. The plasma concentration of lactoferrin, MPO and ECP had already risen after 10min of dialysis and continued steadily to increase during 2h of the dialysis. In contrast to these proteins the increments of lysozyme and lactic dehydrogenase were more modest and not evident until 2h from the start of dialysis.

No difference in the relative increase of the plasma levels of lysozyme was found between the two types of dialyzers used. The increment of lactoferrin, MPO and ECP was, throughout the dialysis, more pronounced with the plate than with the capillary dialyzer, that is more pronounced with the cuprophane membrane.

The intracellular contents of all four granular proteins were reduced after 2h of experimental dialysis. The reduction of the intracellular contents of lactoferrin and lysozyme seemed disproportionate. Extraction of dialysis membranes indicated that lysozyme and lactoferrin in particular were membrane associated.

When performing dialysis with plasma with *added* purified granular proteins or total extracts of granulocyte granules, it was found that these granular proteins adhere to the dialysis membrane, especially lactoferrin and lysozyme, while only about 10% of the added MPO and ECP was bound to the dialyzer.

In order to find out whether serum samples obtained at regular intervals during dialysis were capable of inducing degranulation when added to granulocytes isolated from fresh blood, it was found that no difference in degranulation could be observed in the samples obtained prior to or during the dialysis procedure, nor was there any drop in their total complement of the serum samples.

From the experiments it is obvious that neutrophil and eosinophil degranulation may occur during hemodialysis without having a patient in the circuit. The mechanism whereby this degranulation occurs is uncertain but observed during both plate and capillary dialysis with different membranes. The observed increase in the plasma concentration of granular proteins may reflect a traumatic effect from peristaltic pumping or release from dying granulocytes trapped in the dialyzer. But this is not likely, since the increase of lactoferrin, MPO and ECP was already evident after 10min and the increase of lactic dehydrogenase was very modest and apparent only during the last period of experimental dialysis. Another mechanism may be that plasma requires the capacity to induce granulocyte degranulation. Previous investigators have shown that exposure of plasma to dialyzer membrane may generate activated complement components and at least profound activation of the complement system is associated with degranulation of neutrophils. However, in this study we found no signs of complement activation during experimental dialysis, as measured from CH50 measurements, nor did the serum samples obtained at different times during the dialysis procedure induce an enhanced in vitro degranulation of isolated granulocytes. These findings indicate that plasma is not directly responsible for the degranulation process but that the degranulation occurs by the cellular contact with the dialysis membrane. Only a small proportion of neutrophils remains associated with the dialysis membrane in contrast to the eosinophils which are more apt to be trapped within the dialyzer. This observation is in accordance with the view that early transient neutropenia, observed in patients during hemodialysis, does not reflect cell adhesion to the dialysis membrane but capture of neutrophils in the microvessels, e.g. in the lungs.

Conclusion

The results clearly indicate that the signs of neutrophil and eosinophil degranulation in patients undergoing hemodialysis reflect local degranulation in the dialyzer rather than in the lungs.

References

1 Kaplow, L.S.; Goffinet, J.A.: Profound neutropenia during the early phase of hemodialysis. J. Am. med. Ass. *203*: 1135–1137 (1968).

2 Brubaker, L.H.; Nolph, K.D.: Mechanisms of recovery from neutropenia induced by hemodialysis. Blood *38*: 623–631 (1971).

3 Craddock, P.R.; Fehr, J.; Brigham, K.L.; Kronenberg, R.S.; Jacob, H.S.: Complement and leukocyte-mediated pulmonary dysfunction in hemodialysis, New Engl. J. Med. *296*: 769–774 (1977).

4 Craddock, P.R.; Fehr, J.; Dalmasso, A.P.; Brigham, K.L.; Jacob, H.S.: Hemodialysis leukopenia. Pulmonary vascular leukostasis resulting from complement activation by dialyzer cellophane membranes. J. clin. Invest. *59*: 879–888 (1977).

5 Hällgren, R.; Venge, P.; Wikström, B.: Hemodialysis-induced increase in serum lactoferrin and serum eosinophil cationic protein as signs of local neutrophil and eosinophil degranulation. Nephron *29*: 233–238 (1981).

6 Hällgren, R.; Venge, P.; Danielson, B.G.: Neutrophil and eosinophil degranulation during hemodialysis are mediated by the dialysis membrane. Nephron *32*: 329–334 (1982).

B.G. Danielson, MD, Department of Internal Medicine, University Hospital,
S-75185 Uppsala (Sweden)

Contr. Nephrol., vol. 37, pp. 89–95 (Karger, Basel 1984)

Altered Whole Blood Chemiluminescence during Hemodialysis Using Different Dialysis Membranes

H. Bauer, H. Brunner, B. Spohn, H.E. Franz

Section of Nephrology, University of Ulm, 1st Department of Internal Medicine, Ulm FRG

Introduction

More than 10 years ago a transient leukopenia has been described during hemodialysis using cellulose and cuprophane dialysis membranes [6]. Since that time, biocompatibility of hemodialysis membranes is a widely discussed problem, mainly because today some new membrane materials are available which cause a much less severe leukopenia [1, 9]. Much less is known about changes in leukocyte function during hemodialysis accompanying the decrease in number of white blood cells. An increased adhesiveness of leukocytes has been described in the early phase of hemodialysis [8]. Other tests, like chemotaxis, phagocytosis and aggregation showed conflicting results, possibly caused by artefacts by the isolation of white blood cells [2, 4]. And it is difficult to distinguish between the effects of uremia and of hemodialysis treatment. Chemiluminescence, i.e. light emission during chemical reactions, can be observed when highly reactive radicals like singlet oxygen are formed. During the phagocytosis and killing of bacteria the metabolism of neutrophil granulocytes is activated, the oxygen consumption increases, free radicals are formed and chemiluminescence can be observed. This light emission can be amplified by the addition of luminol and is strongly correlated with the killing of bacteria by leukocytes [5].

Patients and Methods

We performed our study on chronic hemodialysis patients who were dialysed using capillary dialyzers made of either cuprophane (Asahi AM 10) or polymethylmethacrylate (Toray

B2M). For determination of leukocytes and chemiluminescence, 1 ml of blood was drawn from the arterial and venous blood line. Samples were taken before and 15, 30, 60, 120 and 240 min after the beginning of dialysis. 10 units of heparin per ml blood were added for anticoagulation. Leukocyte counts were done in a Coulter counter model ZF and cell differentiation was performed. Whole blood chemiluminescence was measured according to a modification of the method of *Kato* et al. [7]. 50 μl of whole blood were diluted in HBSS buffer. After 10 min incubation with luminol, phagocytes were activated by addition of 20 μl of a standardized suspension of *Escherichia coli*, or by a solution of phorbolmyristate or FMLP, a chemotactic tripeptide. Light emission was determined in a luminometer (Biolumat, Berthold), which has the advantage of an extremely low dark current. We determined the specific chemiluminescence, i.e. the light emission per leukocyte. Besides this, the time course of chemiluminescence of each sample was monitored continuously during at least 30 min. Sample preparation and measurements were done at a temperature of 37 °C.

As a model for mechanical stress for blood cells, we chose the centrifugation of whole blood. Samples taken from healthy volunteers were centrifuged for different times at 2,000 rpm and cells were resuspended afterwards in the original plasma, and chemiluminescence was determined.

Results

During hemodialysis using cuprophane membranes, we saw the well-known leukopenia during the first hour of dialysate, while polymethylmethacrylate (PMMA) showed only a minimal effect on white blood cells.

Maximum Specific Chemiluminescence during Hemodialysis Treatment

Besides the leukopenia, maximum specific chemiluminescence was reduced to 40 ± 14 % of the initial value ($p < 0.001$) 15 min after the start of dialysis using cuprophane membranes. After 60 min, specific chemiluminescence returned to control values (fig. 1).

Comparing the chemiluminescence of blood samples drawn from the arterial and the venous bloodline at the same time, we saw a slight diminution of maximal chemiluminescence of the venous bloodline. But the result was not significant (fig. 1). In contrast to cuprophane, PMMA showed no significant influence on specific chemiluminescence. Samples from the venous bloodline, too, showed a slightly decreased chemiluminescence. There was no statistical significance (fig. 2, 3).

Kinetic of Chemiluminescence during Hemodialysis

Whole blood of healthy persons and uremic patients who have never been dialysed shows a sigmoid time course of light emission after activation

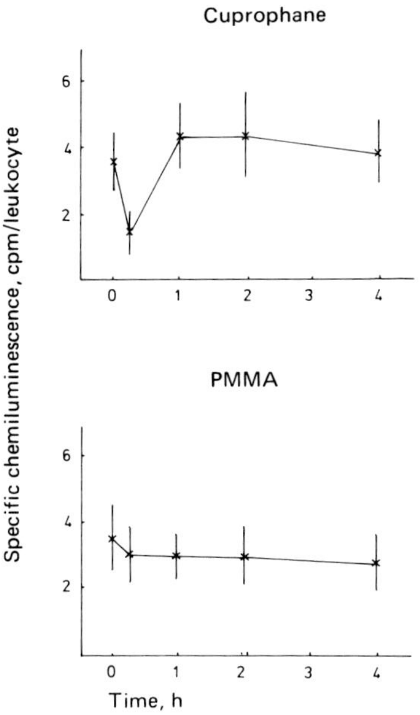

Fig. 1. Specific whole blood chemiluminescence during hemodialysis with cuprophane membranes.

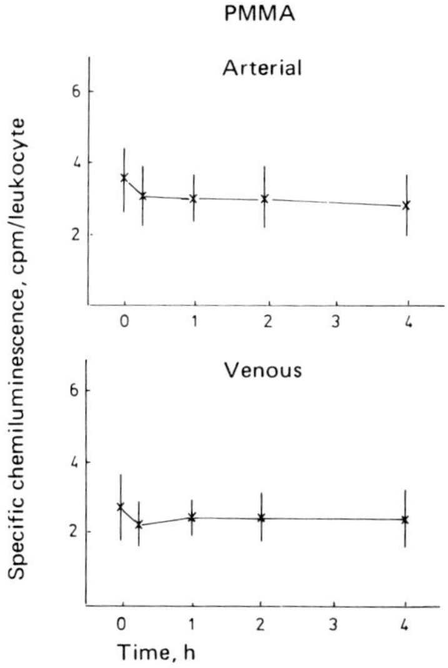

Fig. 2. Specific whole blood chemiluminescence during hemodialysis with PMMA membranes.

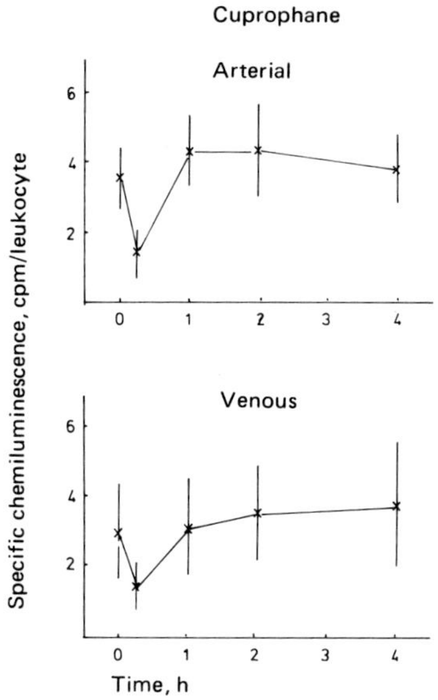

Fig. 3. Comparison of specific whole blood chemiluminescence during hemodialysis with cuprophane and PMMA membranes.

by *E.coli* (fig. 4). After addition of bacteria whole blood shows chemiluminescence after a latent period of about 1–2 min. The maximum light emission is reached after about 15–20 min. Hemodialysis patients show a somewhat different time course of chemiluminescence. The initial increase of light emission after activation is quite faster, the curve loses its sigmoid shape and becomes biphasic in various degrees. A smaller first peak can be seen about 4 min after activation and the second peak occurs as usual after 15–20 min (fig. 5). These changes are more pronounced on the venous blood line and increase towards the end of dialysis. These alterations of the time course of chemiluminescence were independent of the material the dialyzers were made of (fig. 6).

Kinetic of Chemiluminescence after Centrifugation of Whole Blood

Similar effects on the time course of whole blood chemiluminescence as during hemodialysis could be seen when whole blood was centrifuged for several minutes and resuspended afterwards. The curve lost its sigmoid shape and showed a small second peak about 4 min after the activation of leukocytes besides the main peak at 15 min.

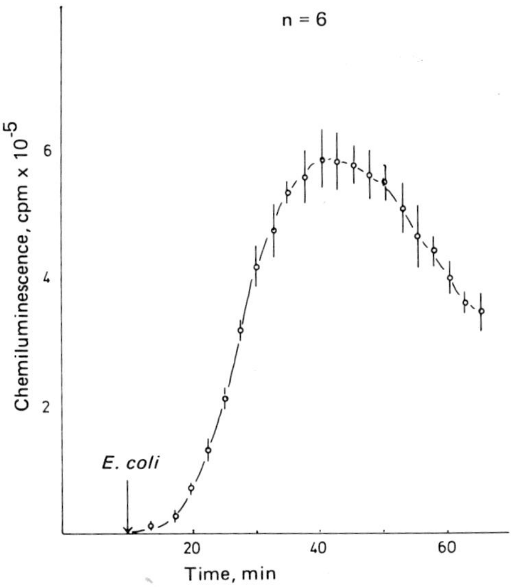

Fig. 4. Whole blood chemiluminescence by simultaneous and discontinuous monitoring of 6 samples.

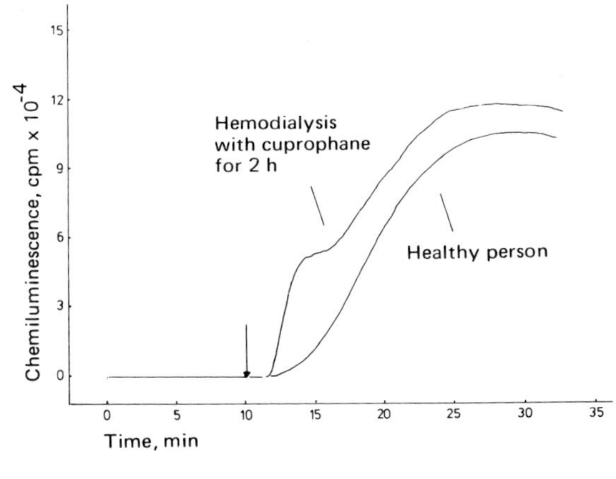

Fig. 5. Whole blood chemiluminescence of a healthy person and a hemodialysis patient (continuous monitoring).

Discussion

Our study shows several effects of cuprophane hemodialyzer membranes on white blood cells: The number of neutrophil granulocytes decreases after 15 min of dialysis. But besides this, the remaining cells in circulation show a diminished chemiluminescence. And because there is a strong correlation between chemiluminescence and bactericidal activity of

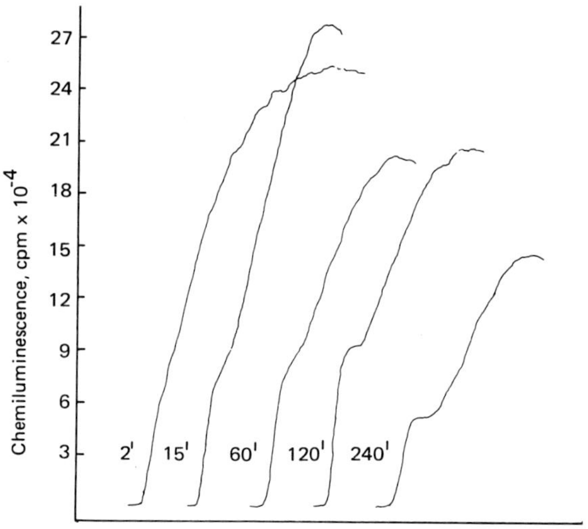

Fig. 6. change of whole blood chemiluminescence kinetics during hemodialysis (PMMA).

leukocytes, this indicates a temporary impairment of antimicrobial defense. The decrease of chemiluminescence occurs at the same time as the activation of the complement system [1, 3] and the increase in adhesiveness of neutrophils [8]. But up to now, little can be said about the relations between these events. The lack of difference in chemiluminescence between blood samples drawn from the arterial and the venous lines indicates that there is no rapid activation or destruction of white blood cells during a single passage through the dialyzer. The activation of neutrophils, which is necessary for the sequestration of cells and the development of leukopenia, seems to be a slow process that needs several minutes and partly occurs in the body and not in the dialyzer. But the single steps of this activation are not known. The small difference in chemiluminescence we observed between blood from the arterial and venous line seems to be caused by the dialysate.

The above-mentioned alterations of the kinetic of chemiluminescence is an additional effect of hemodialysis on white blood cells. Up to now, we do not know the exact mechanisms that determine the shape of the activation curve of whole blood. The loss of the sigmoid curve seems to be caused by the passage of blood through the dialyzer and may reflect a mechanical damage of white blood cells. We assume this, because centrifugation of blood can produce the same effects and there is no difference between the two types of dialyzers we used.

After this study we think that the interaction between hemodialysis membranes and white blood cells is a much more complex problem than had been assumed up to now.

References

1 Aljama, P.; Bird, P.A.E.; Ward, M.K.; Feest, T.G.; Walker, W.; Tanboga, H.; Sussman, M.; Kerr, D.N.S.: Hemodialysis-induced leucopenia and activation of complement: effects of different membranes. Proc. Eur. Dial. Transplant Ass. *15*: 144–153 (1978).

2 Björksten, B.; Mauer, S.M.; Mills, E.L.; Quie, P.G.: The effect of hemodialysis on neurophil chemotactic responsiveness. Acta med. scand. *203*: 67–70 (1978).

3 Craddock, P.R.; Hammerschmid, D.; White, G.; Jacob, H.S.: Complement (C5a–) induced granulocyte aggregation in vitro: a possible mechanism of complement-mediated leukostasis and leukopenia. J. clin. Invest. *60*: 260–264 (1977).

4 Hällgren, R.; Fjellström, K.-E.; Häkansson, L.; Venge, P.: Kinetic studies of phagocytosis. II. The serum-independent uptake of IgG-coated particles by polymorphnuclear leukocytes from uremic patients on regular dialysis treatment. J. Lab. clin. Med. *94*: 277–284 (1979).

5 Horan, T.D.; English, D.; McPherson, A.: Association of neutrophil chemiluminescence with microbicial activity. Clin. Immunopathol. *22*: 259–269 (1982).

6 Kaplow, L.W.; Goffinet, J.A.: Profound neutropenia during the early phase of hemodialysis. J. Am. med. Ass. *203*: 1135–1137 (1968).

7 Kato, T.; Wokalek, H.; Schöpf, E.; Eggert, H.; Ernst, M.; Rietschel, E.T.; Fischer, H.: Measurement of chemiluminescence in freshly drawn human blood. Klin. Wschr. *59*: 203–211 (1981).

8 Lespier-Dexter, L.E.; Guerra, C.; Ojeda, W.; Martinez-Maldonado, M.: Granulocyte adherence in uremia and hemodialysis. Nephron *24*: 64–68 (1979).

9 Shin, J.; Matsuo, M.: Shinko, S.; Fujita, Y.; Inoue, S.; Sakai, R.; Nishioka, M.: A study on hemodialysis leukopenia using various dialyzers. J. Dial. *4*: 51–62 (1980).

H. Bauer, MD, Sektion Nephrologie, Universität Ulm, Steinhövelstrasse 9, D-7900 Ulm/Donau (FRG)

Contr. Nephrol., vol. 37, pp. 96–100 (Karger, Basel 1984)

Biocompatibility of Various Dialysis Membranes as Assessed by Coagulation Assay

M.L. Gasparotto, M. Bertoli, U. Vertolli, A. Ruffatti, M.L. Stoppa, D. Di Landro, G.F. Romagnoli

Sections of Nephrology and Hemodialysis, Padua, Italy

Introduction

It is known that hemodialysis, due to the blood membrane interface, determines adherence of blood cells to the membranes, activation of coagulation and formation of microcoagulums with consumption of coagulation factors [4, 6, 7]. Fibrinolysis is also stimulated simultaneously with clot activation during hemodialysis tending to break up the clots formed [1]. Anticoagulation with heparin, normally used during hemodialysis, does not in fact prevent clot activation since it acts only on the second phase of coagulation. Several studies have shown that clot formation depends markedly on variation in the chemical and geometric structure of the membranes [5].

For this reason, we considered it worthwhile to evaluate some parameters of blood coagulation and fibrinolysis in a group of patients under treatment with different dialysis membranes.

Material and Methods

The study was performed in 10 patients (7 males and 3 females) with an average age of 41 ± 5 years, in maintenance hemodialysis from 6 months to 8 years. All patients had an arteriovenous fistula and were dialyzed for 4h thrice weekly. Blood flow was kept at $300 cm^3$/min, and anticoagulation was obtained by means of continuous heparinization with clotting times ranging from 15 to 20min, (1,500–2,000 U/heparin(h)). None had thromboembolic disease, active infection or evidence of liver disease; none was under treatment with drugs that could alter the results of the tests examined.

The study was conducted using cellulose hydrate membranes (Secon 133, $0.7 m^2$; Secon 104, $1.2 m^2$), cellulose acetate membranes (DAK 4000, $1.2 m^2$), polyacrylonitrile (PAN) membranes (RP 607, $0.67 m^2$) and cuprophan membranes (Gambro 11.5, $1 m^2$).

After a week of treatment with the dialyzers the following dosages were evaluated: platelet and leukocyte (WBC) counts (Automatic Analyzer); fibrinogen level, antithrombin III (AT III), plasminogen and α_1-antitrypsin (radial immunodiffusion); serum fibrinogen degradation products (FDP) (hemagglutininhibition); factor VIII coagulant (F VIII:C) (one time method); factor VIII antigen (F VIII R:Ag) (immunoelectrodiffusion) and fibrinogen half-life (labelled F-^{125}I Takeda technique) [9].

The tests were performed at the beginning and end of each dialysis session from the arterial branch of the fistulas and after 1 h from both arterial and venous branches. Platelets and WBC were tested at 15 min and the fibrinogen half-life at 15, 30, 45, 60 min, 2 and 4 h. The statistical evaluation was made by means of Student's t test.

Results

Platelet and WBC counts diminished rapidly and significantly ($p<0.01$) during the first 15 min of the dialysis with all types of dialyzers except the PAN where the WBC remained stable.

Fibrinogen, plasminogen, AT III and α_1-antitrypsin were within the normal limits at the beginning of dialysis and did not undergo significant modifications at 1 h, nor at the termination of treatment with the four types of membranes. FDP levels, normal before dialysis, rose significantly ($p<0.01$) after 1 h in the venous circuit samples and remained elevated after dialysis with all dialyzers. Coagulant activity of factor VIII, significantly high ($p<0.01$) before dialysis, is usually not doseable at the end. Only 2 patients with very high levels had residual coagulant activity. F VIII R:Ag is also significantly high ($p<0.01$) before dialysis, with few variations during treatment, except when using cuprophan membranes where there was a significant elevation (both absolute and relative to other membranes) at the first hour and at the end of dialysis (table I). Table II shows fibrinogen half-life during hemodialysis. Only Secon 133 presents reduced half-lives compared to other dialyzers.

Discussion

WBC, platelets and fibrinogen half-life diminish during the first minutes of dialysis [3]. As shown in figure 1, fibrinogen half-life was evaluated in each of the various dialyzers using serial blood samples. The results demonstrated a major consumption in the first hour. The increase in FDP is an index of fibrinolysis subsequent to fibrin formation.

The annulment of coagulant activity of factor VIII is a consequence of anticoagulation. High levels of F VIII R:Ag were found at the end of treat-

Table I. Coagulation and fibrinolysis data during dialysis

	Cuprophan (G11.5)		PAN (RP607)		Cellulose Hydrate (Secon 133)		Cellulose acetate (DAK 4000)	
	before	after	before	after	before	after	before	after
Fibrinogen, mg/dl (NV 300 ± 100)	348 ± 98.9	395 ± 50.4	248 ± 54	372 ± 46.2	297 ± 100	379 ± 50.3	350 ± 43.2	380 ± 51.3
FDP, μg/ml (NV 4.9 ± 2.8)	7.5 ± 3.8	69 ± 1.5	8 ± 3.2	51.3 ± 2.2	6.5 ± 5.1	47.5 ± 2.5	8.1 ± 4.3	57.3 ± 10.2
Factor VIII: C, % (NV 94 ± 54.82)	117 ± 33.1	–	105 ± 26.6	–	150 ± 70	–	137 ± 17.5	–
Factor VIII R: Ag, % (NV 81.3 ± 22.86)	179 ± 72.1	537 ± 404.06	191.25 ± 69.35	343.75 ± 156.38	325 ± 172.55	433 ± 162.89	180 ± 20	330 ± 20
AT III, mg/dl (NV 27.13 ± 3.5)	20.56 ± 4.94	22.08 ± 4.33	23.83 ± 7.16	27.95 ± 9.97	32.42 ± 7.34	32.96 ± 4.66	33.41 ± 6.31	31.98 ± 5.62
Plasminogen, mg/dl (NV 10.5 ± 0.93)	8.07 ± 2.30	9.38 ± 2.23	13.18 ± 3.26	14.21 ± 3.13	12.73 ± 2.97	12.51 ± 1.97	13.73 ± 2.91	12.52 ± 1.91
α_1-Antitrypsin mg/dl (NV 300 ± 100)	208.54 ± 66.55	193.99 ± 32.71	200.91 ± 49.96	209.25 ± 15.84	230.25 ± 47.48	241.45 ± 8.16	220.10 ± 41.45	230.22 ± 16.30

NV = Normal values.

Table II. Fibrinogen half-life

	Cuprophan	PAN	Cellulose hydrate		Cellulose acetate
	(G11.5)	(RP607)	Secon 133	Secon 104	(DAK 4000)
$T_{1/2}$, h (NV 93.36 ± 16.08)	3.36 ± 0.27	3.34 ± 0.39	4.68 ± 0.92	3.17 ± 0.04	2.77 ± 0.80

NV = Normal values.

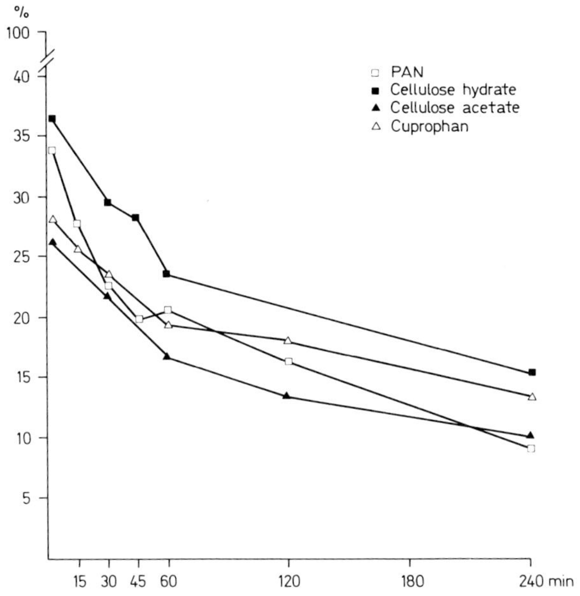

Fig. 1. Percent decrease of labelled fibrinogen-^{125}I during a single hemodialysis session with various dialysis membranes.

ment. This may be due to damage of endothelial cells or platelets with consequent release of F VIII R:Ag [2, 8]. On the other hand, the high basal levels of these two fractions are more difficult to explain.

Plasminogen and α_1-antitrypsin levels do not demonstrate any significant variations. In our opinion, these proteins are not useful for evaluating the fibrinolytic process. If they are consumed they must be rapidly regenerated, but this remains to be demonstrated.

The use of heparin during hemodialysis does not modify AT III levels. As some authors hypothesize [10, 11], this may be due to an antiheparin factor released from platelets or from endothelial release of AT III.

These results are similar for all dialyzers. Using the cellulose hydrate membrane with a surface of $0.75\,m^2$, there is a lower consumption of F-^{125}I, with however, absolute values always increased.

Our study confirms the activation of coagulation with all dialysis membranes. There were no significant differences between the various dialyzers studied.

References

1 Canavese, C.; Stratta, P.; Pacitti, A.; Mangiarotti, G.; Racca, M.; Oneglio, R.; Vercellone, A.: Impaired fibrinolysis in uremia. Partial and variable correction by four different dialysis regimes. Clin. Nephrol. *17*: 82–89 (1982).

2 Howard, M.A.; Whitworth, J.A.; Hendrix, L.E.; Thomas, K.B.; Firkin, B.G.: Abnormal factor VIII in chronic renal failure. Med. J. Aust. *i*: 148–151 (1979).

3 Jacob, A.I.; Gavellas, G.; Zarco, R.; Perez, G.; Bourgoignie, J.J.: Leukopenia, hypoxia, and complement function with different hemodialysis membranes. Kidney int. *18*: 505–509 (1980).

4 Lindsay, R.M.; Prentice, C.R.M.; Davidson, J.F.; Burton, J.A.; McNicol, G.P.: Haemostatic changes during dialysis associated with thrombus formation on dialysis membranes. Br. med. J. *iv*: 454–457 (1972).

5 Lyman, D.J.; Knutson, K.; McNeull, B.; Shibatani, K.: The effects of chemical structure and surface properties of synthetic polymers on the coagulation of blood. Trans. Am. Soc. artif. internal Organs *21*: 49–54 (1975).

6 Marshall, J.W.; Ahearn, D.J.; Nothum, R.J.; Esterly, G.; Nolph, K.D.; Maher, J.F.: Adherence of blood components to dialyzer membranes, morphological studies. Nephron *12*: 157–170 (1974).

7 Mason, R.G.; Shermer, R.W.; Rodman, R.F.: Reaction of blood with nonbiologic surfaces. Am. J. Path. *69*: 271–288 (1972).

8 Remuzzi, G.; Bertani, T.; Mecca, G.; Donati, M.B.; De Gaetano, G.: Factor VIII-related protein on vascular intima of patients with chronic renal failure and prolonged bleeding times. Br. med. J. *i*: 70–72 (1978).

9 Takeda, Y.: Studies of metabolism and distribution of fibrinogen. J. clin. Invest *45*: 103–111 (1966).

10 Turney, J.H.; Fewell, M.; Williams, L.C.; Dodd, N.; Weston, M.J.: Paradoxical behaviour of antithrombin III during hemodialysis and its prevention with prostacyclin. Clin. Nephrol. *17*: 31–35 (1982).

11 Woods, H.F.; Ash, G.; Weston, M.J.; Bunting, S.; Moncada, S.; Vane, J.R.: Prostacyclin can replace heparin in hemodialysis in dogs. Lancet *ii*: 1075–1077 (1978).

Dr. M.L. Gasparotto, Servizio di Nefrologia ed Emodialisi, Ospedale Civile,
Via Giustiniani 1, I-35100 Padova (Italy)

Contr. Nephrol., vol. 37, pp. 101–106 (Karger, Basel 1984)

Leukopenia, Hypoxemia and Complement Activation during a Single Hemoperfusion

R. Perricone, M. Taccone-Gallucci, C. de Carolis, L. Fontana, V. Mazzarella, M. Morosetti, C.U. Casciani

VI° Clinica Medica e V° Patologia Chirurgica, Università di Roma, Italia

Introduction

It has been proposed that hypoxemia occurring during hemodialysis is related to complement activation by the dialysis membranes. This activation leads to the formation of leukocyte microaggregates which embolize the pulmonary vasculature causing arteriovenous shunting, pulmonary oedema and thus hypoxemia [1–3].

Hemoperfusion using a column with activated charcoal for treatment of patients with uremia was described by *Yatzidis* [4] in 1964. The report of leukopenia during a single hemoperfusion [5] led us to determine whether leukopenia, hypoxemia and complement activation occur during the procedure.

Materials and Methods

5 consenting uremic patients on maintenance hemodialysis for an average of 18 months were studied. Primary renal disease included hypertensive nephrosclerosis (n = 1), polycystic kidney disease (n = 1), interstitial nephritis (n = 1) and chronic glomerulonephritis (n = 2). Prior to hemoperfusion patients plasma complement levels were within normal limits. One single hemoperfusion was performed on each patient for a period of 2h using a column containing activated charcoal coated with methacrylate previously washed with 1,000ml of 0.9% saline containing 15,000 IU of heparin. 5min before the institution of hemoperfusion, patient's blood was anticoagulated with 5,000 IU of heparin administered intravenously. During hemoperfusion, blood flow rates were maintained at 200ml/min. For all complement studies, white blood cell (WBC) count and blood gas analysis, blood samples were drawn anaerobically prior to and after 20, 60 and 120min on hemoperfusion from the arterial line. WBC counts, differential white cell counts, determination of acid-base balance and pO_2 were performed with standard techniques.

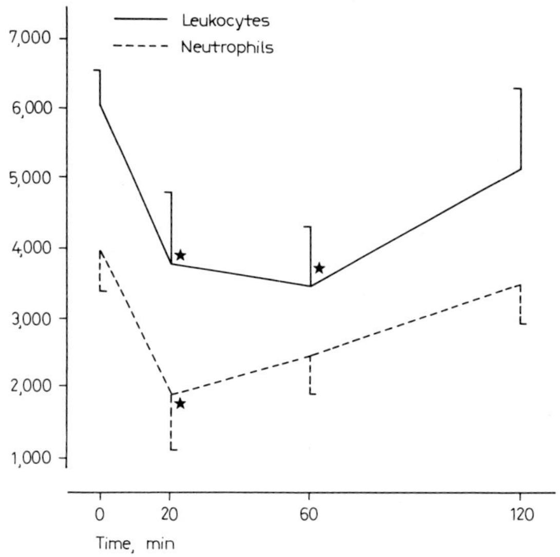

Fig. 1. Mean values ± SD of leukocytes and neutrophils during hemoperfusion. Rapid leukopenia (and neutropenia) occurred within 20min after the initiation of hemoperfusion. $^{*}p<0.02$.

Total hemolytic complement (THC), classical pathway activity (CPA) and alternative pathway activity (APA) were performed as reported previously [6]. The presence of breakdown products from C3 and B was investigated with immunoelectrophoresis [7] in agarose containing EDTA.

Results

In figure 1, the mean values of total WBC (and neutrophils) during hemoperfusion are reported. As can be seen, within 20min after the initiation of hemoperfusion there was a marked drop in WBC count from 6,080 ± 526 to 3,740 ± 1,124 ($p<0.02$); WBC number was still decreased after 60min (3,460 ± 893; $p<0.02$) and raised to 5,200 ± 1,267 at 120min. Prior to hemoperfusion the mean pO_2 value (fig. 2) was 106 ± 13. 8mm Hg. A decrease was observed after 20min (80.2 ± 11.9mm Hg; $p<0.02$) and 60min (77 ± 12.2; $p<0.02$); after 120min, pO_2 tended to increase (87.2 ± 6.2mm Hg).

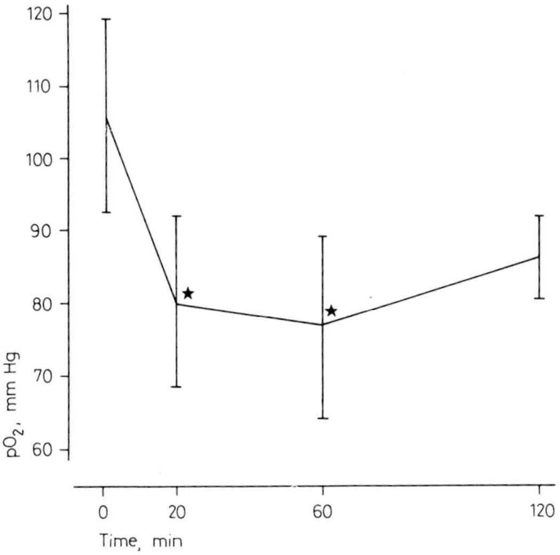

Fig. 2. Mean values ± SD of pO_2 (mm Hg) during hemoperfusion. Within 20 min after the initiation of hemoperfusion, a slight but significant decrease of pO_2 was observed. $^*p<0.02$.

Single regression analysis showed a significant correlation ($r=0.53$; $p<0.05$) among the percent decreases referred to time zero of WBC number and those of pO_2 observed throughout the hemoperfusion period. pH, pCO_2 and HCO_3^- remained constant at all hemoperfusion times. The mean values of THC, CPA and APA during hemoperfusion are reported in figure 3. Within 20 min after the institution of hemoperfusion there was a marked decrease in THC from 135 ± 15.7 to 123 ± 14.7 U/ml ($p<0.001$), in APA from 38.1 ± 5.1 to 33.1 ± 6.7 U/ml ($p<0.005$). After 60 min, the two parameters were still depressed (125 ± 14 U/ml, $p<0.001$ and 30.6 ± 9.7 U/ml, $p<0.05$, respectively). After 120 min THC was 127 ± 14.5 U/ml ($p<0.005$), APA 33.5 ± 7.6 U/ml ($p<0.05$). No significant variation of CPA was observed throughout the study.

Samples of normal human serum or of plasma obtained from one of the patients prior to hemoperfusion were incubated with different concentrations of activated charcoal coated with methacrylate at 37 °C. After 15 and 60 min THC and APA showed a progressive dose-dependent decrease.

All in vivo and in vitro reductions of complement activities were due to a specific activation of the complement system with the formation of complement cleavage fragments as demonstrated by the identification of C3 and B cleavage fragments with the immunoelectrophoretic analysis.

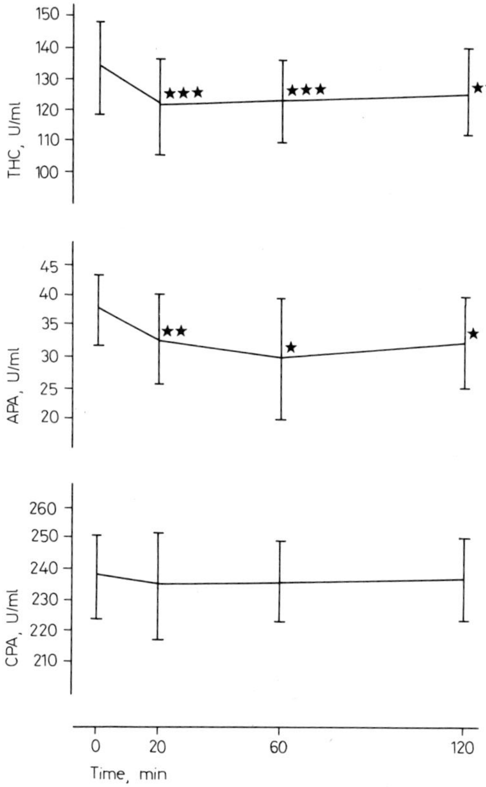

Fig. 3. Changes in THC, APA and CPA during hemoperfusion. Values of hemolytic units per milliliter (U/ml) are expressed as mean ± SD. *$p<0.05$; **$p<0.005$; ***$p<0.001$.

Discussion

Our results demonstrate that leukopenia, hypoxemia and complement activation occur during hemoperfusion. Previous papers showed that dialyzer cuprophan membranes activate complement and that this activation is accompanied, during hemodialysis, by hypoxemia and leukopenia [1–3]. The etiology of the dialysis-related hypoxemia is still a matter of controversy. While *Craddock* et al. [1, 2] suggested the pathogenic sequence complement activation-chemotactic components generation-pulmonary vascular sequestration of leukocytes-hypoxemia, other authors pointed out that a strict correlation in hemodialysis among complement activation, leukopenia and hypoxemia should require that hypoxemia occurs only in patients dialyzed with membranes that cause leukopenia, and gives no account of the progression of hypoxemia during dialysis, despite the release of entrapped pulmonary leukocytes [8, 9].

In hemoperfused patients, the results indicate, on the contrary, a statistically significant correlation between hypoxemia and leukopenia, and that the decrease in pO_2 is transient and lasts no longer than leukopenia.

In hemodialyzed patients, hypoxemia has been alternatively ascribed to a depression of ventilation due to a loss of carbon dioxide across the kidney into the dialysate [10] and to a progressive improvement in acidosis [11].

During hemoperfusion, no loss of CO_2 was recorded (the dialysate was not present in the system) and the pH remained constant at any hemoperfusion time.

Our data show that the degree of complement activation and leukopenia varied over the same time scale, and that maximum leukopenia and maximum complement activation were reached almost simultaneously and lasted no longer than 20–60 min. These findings make it tempting to speculate that complement activation is at least one of the possible mechanisms responsible for leukopenia in this situation. On the other hand, our in vitro experiments clearly demonstrate that charcoal coated with methacrylate is an activator of complement alternative pathway.

The potential clinical significance of complement activation, leukopenia and hypoxemia during hemoperfusion is not clear at all. However, it is conceivable that in high-risk patients, i.e. those with pulmonary diseases, a closer monitoring or routine supplementary oxygen therapy during hemoperfusion will be of benefit.

References

1 Craddock, P.R.; Fehr, S.; Dalmasso, A.P.; Brigham, K.L.; Jacob, H.S.: Hemodialysis leukopenia. Pulmonary vascular leukostasis resulting from complement activation by dialyzer cellophane membranes. J. clin. Invest. *59*: 879–888 (1977).

2 Craddock, P.R.; Fehr, S.; Brigham, K.L.; Kronenberg, R.S.; Jacob, H.S.: Complement and leukocyte-mediated pulmonary dysfunction in hemodialysis. New Engl. J. Med. *296*: 769–774 (1977).

3 De Simone, C.; Perricone, R.; Taccone-Gallucci, M.; Cicogna, V.A.; Rovina, R.; Fontana, L.; Casciani, C.U.: Complement levels in hemodialysis patients (Abstract). VIIth Int. Congr. Nephrology, Montreal 1978.

4 Yatzidis, H.: A convenient hemoperfusion micro-apparatus over charcoal for the treatment of endogenous and exogenous intoxications: its use as an artificial kidney. Proc. Eur. Dial. Transplant Ass. *1*: 83–87 (1964).

5 Ouelès, R.; Asaba, H.; Nelihäuser, M.; Yahiel, V.; Gunnarson, B.; Bergström, J.; Fürst, P.: The removal of uraemic small and middle molecules and free amino acids by carbon hemoperfusion. Trans. Am. Soc. artif. internal Organs *23*: 583–589 (1977).

6 Perricone, R.; De Carolis, C.; De Sanctis, G.; Fontana, L.: Complement activation by cigarette smoke condensate and tobacco infusion. Archs envir. Hlth (in press).

7 Scheidegger, J.J.: Une micro-methode de l'immunoélectrophorèse. Int. Archs Allergy *7*: 103–110 (1955).

8 Bogue, B.A.; Butruille, Y.; Ebert, C.; Gagneux, S.A.; Strom, J.: Absence of cardiopulmonary dysfunction using AN-69 as compared with cellulosic membranes. Proc. Dial. Transplant Forum *1977*: 170–175.

9 Mahajan, S.; Gardiner, H.; Detor, B.; Desai, S.; Muller, B.; Johnson, N.; Briggs, W.; McDonald, F.: Relationships between pulmonary functions and hemodialysis induced leukopenia. Trans. Am. Soc. artif. internal Organs *23*: 411–415 (1977).

10 Sherlock, J.; Ledwith, J.; Letteri, J.: Hypoventilation and hypoxemia during hemodialysis: reflex response to removal of CO_2 across the dialyzer. Trans. Am. Soc. artif. internal Organs *23*: 406–410 (1977).

11 Jacob, A.I.; Gavellas, G.; Zarco, R.; Perez, G.; Bourgoigne, J.J.: Leukopenia, hypoxia and complement function with different hemodialysis membranes. Kidney int. *18*: 505–509 (1980).

Dr. R. Perricone, Clinica Medica VI, University of Rome, Policlinico Umberto I,
Viale del Policlinico, I-00161 Rome (Italy)

Contr. Nephrol., vol. 37, pp. 107–110 (Karger, Basel 1984)

Dialysis Hypoxemia: The Role of Fibronectin and Its Pathophysiological Implication

H.P. Schwarz, H. Graf, A. Luger, J. Kovarik, H.K. Stummvoll
2nd Department of Medicine, University Clinic of Vienna, Austria

Introduction

Transient hypoxemia during the initial phase of hemodialysis (HD) has been primarily observed by *Johnson* et al. [1]. Studies in the experimental animal suggested that plasma contact with cellulose membranes results in complement activation and a subsequent sequestration of granulocytes in the pulmonary vasculature [2]. Previous reports from our group confirmed this finding in man [3] and suggested that complement-mediated leukostasis leads to an acute pulmonary dysfunction as the causative event of dialysis hypoxemia [4].

Fibronectin, a high molecular weight glycoprotein, is present in a soluble form in blood and in an insoluble form in tissue. It takes part in a great variety of physiological processes such as coagulation, fibrinolysis and opsonization [5]. Besides, it seems to play a major role in the maintenance of cellular and extracellular integrity [6].

Acute depletion of plasma fibronectin has been reported in the adult respiratory distress syndrome (ARDS) [7], in the critically ill patient [8], and following trauma. Since ARDS and dialysis hypoxemia show striking similarities it seemed of interest to investigate the behavior of plasma fibronectin during HD [9].

Patients, Methods and Results

6 patients (3 males, 3 females) with chronic renal failure under intermittent hemodialysis using cellulosic membranes (C-DAK, Cordis Dow, dialysis membrane surface 1.8 or 2.5 m^2) were studied. Blood was drawn from the 'arterial' site of the av fistula at 0, 10, 20, 30, 40, 50

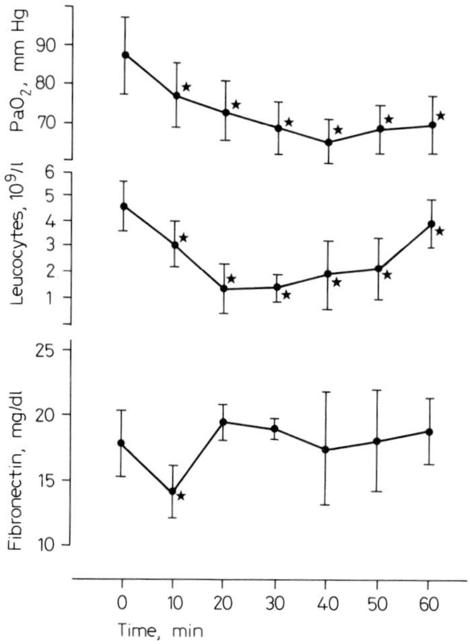

Fig. 1. Fibronectin levels (mean ± SEM) during the first hour of hemodialysis. *p=<0.02.

and 60min and analyzed for granulocyte count, paO_2, and fibronectin. For fibronectin analysis 9 parts of blood, collected by venipuncture, were drawn into 1 part of 3.8% sodium citrate. After centrifugation for 15min at 2,500rpm, plasma was stored at −30°C in small aliquots. Fibronectin determination was performed by the recently developed immuno-video-nephelometer system [10] using anti-human fibronectin antibodies commercially available (Behringwerke). Granulocytes dropped significantly 10min after the start of HD, being accompanied by the well-known drop of paO_2.

Fibronectin also dropped significantly after 10min, the curves of all three parameters showing an almost identical shape during the whole observation period (fig. 1).

Discussion

Our results show that fibronectin levels drop concomitantly to the occurrence of hypoxemia and granulocytopenia in the early phase of HD using cellulosic dialyzer membranes. Experimental and clinical evidence has accumulated, implicating complement-mediated neutrophil aggregation and stasis in pulmonary capillaries in the genesis of pulmonary endothelial injury that characterizes ARDS [9]. Transient neutropenia occurring during HD is the result of neutrophil aggregation and deposition in pulmonary vessels during the neutropenic interval, as has been shown by *Craddock* et al. [2].

Neutrophils produce proteases that destroy structural proteins such as collagen, elastin and fibronectin [11]. Thus, the drop in fibronectin as shown in our data could be due to a destruction of fibronectin by increased neutrophil protease activity released by entrapped leucocytes, a phenomenon implicated in the genesis of ARDS.

Depletion of fibronectin, a major serum opsonin, results in a depression of the phagocytic function of the reticuloendothelial system [12]. Reticuloendothelial system failure leads to prolonged circulation of blood-born microparticles and products of disseminated coagulation which enhance injuries on the pulmonary endothelium [13]. As a result an increased extrahepatic uptake especially in the lungs takes place. Reticuloendothelial system dysfunction therefore may result in microembolization of pulmonary vessel walls and increased permeability of the endothelium resulting in alterations in fluid exchange, and disrupted gas exchange mechanisms [14]. On the other hand, tissue-bound fibronectin appears to be of importance in maintaining the integrity of the endothelial surface. If fibronectin deficiency may be associated with elaboration of the protein from vascular endothelial surfaces or release reaction from injured ischemic endothelial cells, this could result in loss of vascular endothelial integrity and increased microvascular permeability.

In conclusion the etiology of dialysis hypoxemia could be explained in the following way. Blood-membrane contact leads to complement activation with sequestration of polymorphonuclear cells in the pulmonary vasculature. Proteases are released from these activated cells and destroy structural proteins such as fibronectin, thus leading to reticuloendothelial system dysfunction and altered pulmonary cellular integrity resulting in an overt disturbance of pulmonary function.

References

1 Johnson, N.R.; Bischel, M.D.; Boylen, C.T.: Hypoxemia and hyperventilation in chronic hemodialysis. Clin. Res. *19*: 145 (1970).

2 Craddock, P.R.; Fehr, J.; Brigham, K.L.; Kronenberg, R.S.; Jacob, H.S.: Complement and leucocyte-mediated pulmonary dysfunction in hemodialysis. New Engl. J. Med. *296*: 769–774 (1977).

3 Stummvoll, H.K.; Graf, H.; Wolf, A.; Leithner, C.: Dialysis-membrane-blood interaction; in Winter, Gibbons, Plenk, Biomaterials 1980, pp. 505–510 (Wiley & Sons, 1982).
4 Graf, H.; Stummvoll, H.K.; Haber, P.; Kovarik, J.: Pathophysiology of dialysis related hypoxemia. Proc EDTA *17*: 155–161 (1980).
5 Mosher, D.F.: Fibronectin; in Spaet, Progress in hemostasis and thrombosis, vol. 5, pp. 111–151 (Grune & Stratton, New York 1980).
6 Rennard, S.T.I.; Crystal, R.G.: Fibronectin in bronchopulmonary lavage fluid. J. clin. Invest. *69*: 113–122 (1981).
7 Saba, T.M.; Blumenstock, F.A.; Scouill, W.A.; Bernhard, H.: Cryoprecipitate reversal of opsonic α_2-surface-binding glycoprotein deficiency in septic surgical and trauma patients. Science *201*: 622–624 (1978).
8 Mosher, D.F.; Williams, E.M.: Fibronectin concentration is decreased in plasma of severely ill patients with disseminated intravascular coagulation. J. Lab. clin. Med. *91*: 729–35 (1978).
9 Rinaldo, J.E.; Rogers, R.M.: Adult respiratory distress syndrome. New Engl. J. Med. *306*: 900–909 (1982).
10 Wider, G.; Kulnigg, E.; Molinari, E.; Hotschek, H.; Bayer, R.M.: Evaluation of a monitor guided nephelometric system. J. clin. Chem. clin. Biochem. *20*: 1–8 (1982).
11 McDonald, J.A.; Baum, B.J.; Rosenberg, D.M.; Kelman, J.A.; Brin, S.C.; Crystal, R.G.: Destruction of a major extracellular adhesive glycoprotein (fibronectin) of human fibrolasts by neutral proteases from polymorphonuclear leucocyte granules. Lab. Invest. *40*: 350–357 (1979).
12 Saba, T.M.; Luzio, N.R.: Retoculoendothelial blockade and recovery as a function of opsonic activity. Am. J. Physiol. *216*: 197–205 (1969).
13 Hyers, T.M.: Pathogenes of adult respiratory distress syndrome: current concepts. Semin. respir. Med. *2*: 104–108 (1981).
14 Saba, T.M.; Cho, E.: Reticuloendothelial systemic response to operative trauma as influenced by cryoprecipitate or cold-insoluble globulin therapy. J. reticuloendoth. Soc. *26*: 171–186 (1979).

H.P. Schwarz, MD, 2nd Department of Medicine, University Clinic of Vienna, Garnisonsgasse 13, A-1090 Vienna (Austria)

Round Table Discussion

Contr. Nephrol., vol. 37, pp. 111–119 (Karger, Basel 1984)

Comparison of Four Dialyzer-Dialysate Combinations: Effects on Blood Gases, Cell Counts, Complement Contact Factors and Fibrinolytic System

N.D. Vaziri, C.H. Barton, A. Warner, J. Toohey, C. Lintner, E. Hung, P. Mullin, B. Samiminia, M. O'Donnell, K. Mallot

Division of Nephrology, University of California, Irvine, Calif., USA

Introduction

Leukopenia and hypoxia are well-recognized complications of hemodialysis [1–3]. These abnormalities have been etiologically linked to the chemical nature of the dialyzer membrane and the composition of dialysate. Earlier studies have suggested possible activation of Hageman factor during dialysis [4]. Activation of Hageman factor is known to result in not only the initiation of intrinsic coagulation pathway but also triggering of kallikrein-kinin system as well as fibrinolytic pathway [5]. The latter can in turn activate complement cascade [1, 2]. Since dialysis leukopenia is thought to be complement mediated [1, 2] we sought to investigate possible activation of Hageman factor during dialysis and its possible link with leukopenia and other dialysis-associated phenomena. In addition, the study was intended to compare the changes of arterial oxygen tension (PO_2) during dialysis with four major dialyzer/dialysate combinations.

Patients, Materials and Methods

Patients. 20 stable patients (11 men and 9 women, aged 23–73 years) with end-stage renal disease (ESRD) were included in the study. They had been maintained on hemodialysis for periods ranging from 3 months to over 10 years. Patients were dialyzed for 4h thrice weekly. Patients with discernible pulmonary, hepatic and coagulation abnormalities were excluded.

Dialysis Experiments. The studies were performed using four different combinations of two dialyzers and two dialysates. The two dialyzers were those made of polyacrylonitrile (PAN, AN69 Hospal) and cuprophan (C). The two dialysates used were acetate-buffered (Ac) and bicarbonate-buffered (Bi) solutions. The former contained $Na^{+} = 138$, Cl^{-} = 103, $CH_3-COO^{-} = 39.5$, $Ca^{++} = 3.5$, $Mg^{++} = 1.0$ and $K^{+} = 0-3$ mEq/l, while the latter contained $Na = 139$, $Cl^{-} = 103.5$, $HCO_3^{-} = 40$, $Ca^{++} = 3.5$, $Mg^{++} = 1.0$ and $K = 0-3$ mEq/l. Anticoagulation was accomplished using systemic heparinization. Dialysate flow rate was 500 ml/min while blood flow rate was 150–200 ml/min. A proportioning bicarbonate dialysate delivery system was used.

Patients were randomly assigned to one of the four dialyzer/dialysate combinations which included C-Ac, PAN-Ac, C-Bi and PAN-Bi. Some patients participated in more than one study.

Analytical Methods. Samples for arterial blood gas analysis were anaerobically collected in heparinized glass syringes and immediately tested using standard methods. Arterial blood gas data were obtained immediately before and 1 h after the onset of dialysis. Blood samples for white blood cell (WBC) count, platelet count and hematocrit were obtained from the arterial line of the dialyzer immediately before dialysis and at 15 min, 30 min, and 1, 2 and 4 h after the onset of dialysis. Simultaneous samples were obtained from the outgoing line of the dialyzer at 30 min. The samples were collected in siliconized EDTA glass tubes and were tested using the standard laboratory methods.

Blood samples for Hageman factor and factor XI assays were collected in plastic tubes containing sodium citrate solution (blood/citrate = 9/1 volume). The samples were immediately centrifuged (at 4 °C for 10 min at $10^3 g$) with plasma separated and immediately snap frozen in liquid nitrogen and stored at −70 °C till assayed. Additional blood samples were obtained for determination of fibrinogen, plasminogen, fibrinogen degradation products (FDP), high molecular weight kininogen (HMK) and C_3 complement levels. Arterial blood samples for these assays were obtained from the arterial line of the dialyzer, immediately before and at 15 min and 4 h after the onset of dialysis. In addition, simultaneous samples were obtained from the outgoing line of the dialyzer at 15 min.

Factors XII and XI procoagulant activities were measured by a modified partial thromboplastin time [6] using congenitally deficient plasmas as substrate. Factor XII concentration was measured by a sensitive rocket immunoelectrophoresis developed in our laboratory using a monospecific antiserum raised in goat against human Hageman factor. A similar method was employed to measure HMK using antiserum against HMK.

Fibrinogen was determined using a turbidimetric method as described by *Cannarzzi* et al. [7]. FDP levels were measured using an agglutination test employing a suspension of latex particles coated with antisera against all D and E fragments purchased from Wellcome Reagents Ltd. (Wellcome Research Laboratories, Beckenham, England). Plasminogen was quantitated using Calbiochem-Behring radial immunodiffusion M-partigen plasminogen kit (purchased from Calbiochem-Behring Corp.). C_3 complement levels were measured using Immuno-plate III Radial Immunodiffusion test kit purchased from Hyland Diagnostic Laboratories, Division of Travenol Laboratories. Paired t test, analysis of the variance and linear regression were used as appropriate. The data are expressed as mean ± SD.

Results

Effects on Arterial PO_2, PCO_2, pH and Bicarbonate (table I). A significant fall in PO_2 was noted when acetate-based dialysate was used. The reduction in PO_2 was more profound with cellulosic membrane than the PAN membrane. No significant change was noted in pH, PCO_2 and bicarbonate after 1h of dialysis with Ac-PAN. Similarly, no significant change was observed in pH and bicarbonate levels with Ac-C, however, a significant rise in PCO_2 was noted.

The mean PO_2 rose slightly with Bi-PAN and fell slightly with Bi-C. These changes, however, did not attain statistical significance. No significant changes were observed in PCO_2 or bicarbonate levels after 1h of dialysis with bicarbonate dialysis with either membrane.

Changes of PCV, WBC and Platelet Counts (table II). With the cellulosic dialyzers WBC count fell significantly within 15min and returned or exceeded the baseline by 60min. Single passage through the dialyzer had no effect on the WBC count. Similarly, the composition of dialysate seemed to have no influence on WBC changes during dialysis. With PAN dialyzers WBC remained virtually unchanged throughout dialysis and on single passage through the dialyzer.

Effects on Factors XII, XI and HMK Levels. Pre- and postdialysis factor XII-act were 95 ± 31 and 94 ± 28%, respectively ($p = NS$) when cellulosic dialyzers were used. The respective values for PAN dialyzers were 97 ± 24 and 94 ± 32% representing no significant difference with dialysis. Factor XII-conc in the group treated with cellulosic dialyzers was $24 \pm$ μg/ml before and 27 ± 9 μg/ml after dialysis ($p = NS$). The respective values in the group dialyzed with PAN dialyzers were 26 ± 7.8 and 28 ± 13.6 μg/ml, respectively ($p = NS$). No significant changes were noted in HMK concentration and factor XI-act during dialysis with either dialyzers. Similarly, no significant changes were observed in factor XII-act, factor XII-conc, factor XI-act or HMK on single passage through neither types of the dialyzers (table III).

Effects on Plasminogen, Fibrinogen and FDP. No significant difference was found in plasminogen concentration during dialysis or on single passage through the dialyzer with neither the cellulosic nor PAN dialyzers. Similarly, no significant change was noted in fibrinogen concentration dur-

Table I. Changes of arterial O_2 tension (P_aO_2), $PaCO_2$, pH and bicarbonate during dialysis with cellulosic (C) and polyacrylonitrile (PAN) membranes and acetate (Ac) and bicarbonate (Bi) dialysates

	PaO_2, mm Hg		$PaCO_2$, mm Hg		pH, units		Bicarbonate, mEq/l	
	0	1 h	0	1 h	0	1 h	0	1 h
C-Ac (n = 5)	108.6 ± 14.8 ($p < 0.02$)	88.6 ± 11.2	24.2 ± 4.2 ($p < 0.01$)	29.0 ± 3.8	7.40 ± 0.10 (NS)	7.37 ± 0.03	14.4 ± 2.6 (NS)	15.9 ± 1.1
C-Bi (n = 5)	123.0 ± 4.9 (NS)	116.9 ± 8.6	32.1 ± 4.4 (NS)	31.9 ± 3.6	7.34 ± 0.05 ($p < 0.01$)	7.4 ± 0.04	16.6 ± 1.4 (NS)	19.0 ± 2.6
PAN-Ac (n = 7)	116.5 ± 11.0 ($p < 0.02$)	104.9 ± 14.6	31.9 ± 6.1 (NS)	33.6 ± 6.1	7.34 ± 0.04 (NS)	7.34 ± 0.04	16.7 ± 4.0 (NS)	17.3 ± 3.0
PAN-Bi (n = 7)	106.3 ± 15.3 (NS)	114.4 ± 11.0	30.7 ± 6.8 (NS)	31.6 ± 2.7	7.30 ± 0.07 (NS)	7.35 ± 0.08	15.1 ± 3.4 (NS)	17.1 ± 3.0

Table II. Changes of WBC count during dialysis with cellulosic and PAN dialyzer and acetate (Ac) and bicarbonates (NI) dialysates

Collection time	0	15 min A	15 min V	30 min	1 h	2 h	4 h
Cellulosic dialyzers							
Ac	8,816 ± 2,798	4,652* ± 1,740	4,604* ± 1,875	5,958* ± 2,051	9,699 ± 2,887	10,219 ± 3,171	9,798 ± 2,083
Bi	5,921 ± 2,200	2,375* ± 1,744	2,709* ± 1,881	5,026 ± 3,377	6,192 ± 3,020	6,796 ± 2,443	6,966 ± 2,606
PAN dialyzers							
Ac	4,832 ± 1,414	4,559 ± 1,191	4,453 ± 1,450	4,836 ± 1,287	5,033 ± 1,270	5,156 ± 1,716	4,529 ± 1,508
Bi	5,156 ± 2,047	4,229 ± 2,010	4,182 ± 2,069	3,903 ± 2,428	4,152 ± 2,008	5,138 ± 1,235	5,604 ± 1,537

*$p<0.05$.

ing dialysis with either dialyzers. A significant rise in FDP from 11.2 ± 6.5 to 25.0 ± 17.3 μg/ml ($p<0.01$) was noted during dialysis with cellulosic dialyzers. The respective values obtained during dialysis with PAN dialyzers (11.4 ± 10.3 and 11.4 ± 12 μg/ml) were virtually identical.

Effect on C_3 Concentration. No significant change was observed in C_3 levels during dialysis or on single passage through neither types of the dialyzers.

Table III. Plasma procoagulant activities (act) of factors XII and XI and concentrations (conc) of factor XII, high molecular weight kininogen (HMK), fibrinogen, plasminogen, fibrinogen degradation products (FDP) and C_3 complement levels before (B) and after (A) dialysis

	PAN dialyzer		Cellulosic dialyzers	
	B	A	B	A
Factor XII-act, % control	97 ± 24	94 ± 32	95 ± 31	94 ± 28
Factor XII-conc, µg/ml	26 ± 7	28 ± 13	24 ± 7	27 ± 9
Factor XI-act, % control	123 ± 24	115 ± 31	131 ± 26	136 ± 40
HMK, % control	131 ± 38	136 ± 48	127 ± 34	150 ± 42
Fibrinogen, mg/dl	329 ± 158	331 ± 84	244 ± 83	254 ± 105
Plasminogen, mg/dl	10.0 ± 3.0	10.4 ± 2.4	7.7 ± 2.1	8.0 ± 2.0
FDP, µg/ml	11.4 ± 10.3	11.4 ± 12.0	11.2 ± 6.5	25.0 ± 17.3*
C_3, mg/dl	120 ± 48	139 ± 54	113 ± 41	108 ± 41

*$p<0.01$.

Discussion

Based on our results, dialysis hypoxia is primarily a function of the dialysate composition, although the type of dialyzer also seems to play a role. Since the main difference between the two dialysates was in their buffer content, it appears that dialysis hypoxia is somehow caused by presence of acetate and prevented or reduced by presence of bicarbonate in the dialysate. Occurrence of hypoxia during acetate dialysis has been previously demonstrated [8–11]. It has been variably attributed to increased O_2 consumption necessitated by acetate metabolism, hypoventilation caused by dialyzer CO_2 losses or a direct effect. While unanimity exists as to the occurrence of hypoxia during conventional acetate dialysis, considerable controversy remains on the effect of bicarbonate dialysis. Bicarbonate dialysis has been shown to produce no hypoxia [12–14], mild hypoxia [15, 16] or marked hypoxia comparable to that of acetate dialysis [11]. The interpretation of these results is made difficult by the marked methodological variations in the study designs. For instance the baths were gassed with CO_2 in some studies, thereby possibility of net transdialyzer CO_2 gain and associated hyperventilation. Other studies had employed glucose-containing dialysate [11] which could have altered O_2 consumption, CO_2 production and respiratory quotient thereby PO_2 due to transdialyzer influx and metabolism of glucose. Moreover, different dialyzers had been used in these studies. In the present study a glucose-free bicarbonate dialysate, instantaneously produced and delivered by a proportioning system, was used. This can preclude the marked intradialytic changes in bicarbonate concentration, commonly experienced with other systems. Using the same bicarbonate dialysate and delivery system, PO_2 showed a mild reduction with cellulosic dialyzers and a mild rise with PAN dialyzers. Similarly the degree of hypoxia with acetate bath was more severe with cuprophan than PAN dialyzer. This observation points to the partial role of dialyzer in the expression of dialysis hypoxia. Our data indicate that in contrast to PAN dialyzers, cuprophan dialyzers tend to potentiate dialysis hypoxia. The observed mild increase in PO_2 with PAN-Bi probably represents improved pulmonary gas exchange associated with ultrafiltration and the resultant decrease in predialysis fluid overload.

The observed leukopenia during dialysis with cuprophan dialyzers irrespective of the dialysate composition is consistent with earlier reports [1, 2]. Similarly, lack of leukopenia during dialysis with PAN dialyzers is in agreement with previous observations [17]. C_3 complement levels showed a mild reduction both on single passage of blood and during dialysis with cuprophan dialyzers. The changes however, did not attain statistical significance. The observed fall in C_3 is consistent with the earlier observations [1, 2] and occurrence of leukopenia in our patients.

Hageman factor concentration and activity showed no significant change both on single passage of blood and during dialysis with either types of dialyzers. Our findings contrast those of an early report by *Wardle and Piercy* [4] demonstrating a significant reduction in factor XII activity during dialysis. The reason for the observed disparity between the two reports is not clear. However, several major methodological differences were evident. In studies reported by *Wardle and Piercy* [4] factor XII procoagulant assay had been performed using a two-stage method employing lysosome-treated plasma (to inhibit factor XII) as substrate. The present study, however, employed a one-stage PTT using congenitally factor XII-deficient plasma as substrate. In addition, a special anion exchange column was used in the present study to remove residual heparin prior to FXII assay. No measures, however, were taken to deal with residual circulating heparin in post-dialysis blood samples in the study by *Wardle and Piercy* [4]. Consequently the apparent postdialysis fall in factor XII reported by these authors could have been due to the effect of residual heparin rather than true factor XII deficiency. It should be noted, however, that lack of significant change in the concentration or activity of factor XII and its closely related factors (factor XI and HMK) in our patients during dialysis does not necessarily preclude activation and consumption of these factors. Continued synthesis and altered intravascular distribution volume associated with ultrafiltration could have potentially masked the effects of a low-grade consumption on plasma concentration of these proteins. To assess these possibilities, we are currently conducting a series of in vitro studies in which no fluid shifts occurs and continued synthesis is obviously nonexistent.

The observed rise in FDP during dialysis with cuprophan dialyzers is indicative of increased fibrinolytic activity. The available data do not allow satisfactory explanation for this phenomenon.

References

1 Craddock, P.R.; Fehr, J.; Brigham, K.L.; Kronenberg, R.S.; Jacob, H.S.: Complement and leukocyte mediated pulmonary dysfunction in hemodialysis. New Engl. J. Med. *296*: 769–744 (1977).

2 Craddock, P.R.; Fehr, J.; Dalmasso, A.P.; Brigham, K.L.; Jacob, H.S.: Hemodialysis leukopenia-pulmonary vascular leukostasis resulting from complement activation by dialyzer cellophane membranes. J. clin. Invest. *59*: 879–888 (1977).

3 Vaziri, N.D.: Dialysis-induced hypoxemia. Int. J. artif. Organs *5*: 8–10 (1982).

4 Wardle, E.N.; Piercy, D.A.: Studies of contact activation of blood in haemodialysis. J. clin. Path. *25*: 1045–1049 (1972).

5 Murano, G.: The Hageman connection: interrelationships of blood coagulation, fibrino(geno)lysis, kinin generation and complement activation. Am. J. Hematol. *4*: 409–417 (1978).

6 Proctor, R.R.; Rappaport, S.I.: The partial thromboplastin time with kaolin. A simple screening test for first stage plasma clotting factor deficiencies. Am. J. clin. Path. *36*: 212 (1961).

7 Cannarzzi, D.B.; Wardlow, S.C.; McPhedran, P.: An improved turbidimetric method for plasma fibrinogen. Am. J. med. Technol. *43*: 211–215 (1977).

8 Patterson, R.W.; Nissenson, A.R.; Miller, J.; Smith, R.T.; Narins, R.G.; Sullivan, S.F.: Hypoxemia and pulmonary gas exchange during hemodialysis. J. appl. Physiol. *50*: 259–264 (1981).

9 Sherlock, J.; Ledwith, J.; Letteri, J.: Hypoventilation and hypoxemia during hemodialysis: reflex response to removal of CO_2 across the dialyzer. Trans. Am. Soc. artif. internal Organs *29*: 406–410 (1977).
10 Dulmer, F.; Levin, N.W.: Leukopenia and hypoxemia unrelated effects of hemodialysis. Archs intern. Med. *139*: 1103–1106 (1979).
11 Eiser, A.R.; et al.: Contrasting alterations in pulmonary gas exchange during acetate and bicarbonate hemodialysis. Am. J. Nephrol. *2*: 123–127 (1982).
12 Nissenson, A.R.: Prevention of dialysis-induced hypoxemia by bicarbonate dialysis. Trans. Am. Soc. artif. internal Organs. *26*: 339–342 (1980).
13 Kroute, J.A.; Grafter, U.; Miller, J.H.; Shinaberger, J.H.: Prevention of arterial hypoxemia during dialysis by use of bicarbonate dialysate. Kidney int. *14*: 678 (1978).
14 Dolan, M.; Whipp, B.; Davidson, W.; Weitzman, R.; Wasserman, K.: Hypopnea associated with acetate hemodialysis: carbon dioxide flow dependent ventilation. New Engl. J. Med. *305*: 72–75 (1981).
15 Abu-Hamdan, D.; Mahajan, S.; Desai, S.; Choi, C.; Mueller, B.; Briggs, W.; McDonald, F.: Hypoxemia during bicarbonate dialysis. Kidney int. *19*: 140 (1981).
16 Gotch, F.; Discussion of dialysis-induced hypoxemia. Trans. Am. Soc. artif. internal Organs *26*: 342 (1980).
17 Shin, J.; Matsuo, M.; Shinko, S.; Fujita, Y.; Inoue, S.; Sakai, R.; Nishioka, M.: A study on hemodialysis leukopenia using various dialyzers. J. Dialysis *4*: 51–62 (1980).

N.D. Vaziri, MD, Room C351, Medical Sciences I, Division of Nephrology, Department of Medicine, University of California, Irvine, CA 92727 (USA)

Contr. Nephrol., vol. 37, pp. 120–128 (Karger, Basel 1984)

Haemodialysis Leucopenia: The Role of Membrane Type and Re-use

N.A. Hoenich, S.R.D. Johnston, C. Woffindin, D.N.S. Kerr
Department of Medicine, University of Newcastle upon Tyne, UK

Introduction

A transient and rapidly reversible fall in white cell count during haemodialysis (haemodialysis leucopenia) was first described by *Kaplow and Goffinet* [13]. This fall and subsequent return to predialysis level, which in some cases is associated with a rebound leucocytosis, occurs within the first hour of each dialysis and has its nadir between 10 and 30min [4, 9, 12]. Differential white cell counts carried out during this phenomenon show that the leucopenia is due to a fall in neutrophils, monocytes and eosinophils which occurs over the same time span as the leucopenia [4, 6, 9, 15].

Initially, clinicians accepted this phenomenon as a feature of regular haemodialysis treatment without much comment, probably for two reasons:

(1) The original authors stated that – 'the transient neutropenia induced by haemodialysis is the most rapid and profound yet reported in man, and is without symptoms or apparent clinical sequelae'.

(2) Haemodialysis membranes, which were recognised as the cause of leucopenia, were then almost exclusively derived from cellulose and most were manufactured in a single factory by the cuprammonium process. There was, therefore, little opportunity to modify the phenomenon and observe the results.

A recent resurgence of interest in leucopenia dates from a series of papers by *Craddock* et al.[5, 6] who described a possible mechanism for leucopenia and suggested that the hypoxia of dialysis was caused by pulmonary dysfunction secondary to the accumulation of leucocytes in the lung capillaries, a suggestion that has not been universally accepted [2, 3, 8]. By this time, other haemodialysis membranes were available and it was possible to study haemodialysis with and without profound leucopenia and to make some assessment of its contribution through symptoms within the limitations imposed by the other differences between the membranes.

We have compared the degree of leucopenia generated by cellulose membranes manufactured by different processes and by synthetic membranes and have investigated the influence of haemodialysis reuse, a factor known to modify leucopenia [9, 11, 15, 18]

Materials and Methods

Subjects

A number of studies, ranging from 4 to 10, were performed on patients receiving three times weekly maintenance haemodialysis. Ethical committee approval and patient consent was obtained for all studies. The patients who co-operated in the study were randomly allocated to the membranes studied from our dialysis population. All patients had arteriovenous fistulas, used acetate-containing haemodialysis concentrate, were free from infection and were taking no drugs known to affect white cell count.

Materials

Modified cellulose membranes, manufactured by the Cordis Dow Corporation (Cellulate®, and Saponified Cellulose Ester; SCE) and synthetic membranes manufactured by Hospal, (Lyons, France) (AN 69S), Asahi Medical Co. Ltd. (Tokyo, Japan) (PAN 15), Gambro (Lund, Sweden) (Polycarbonate; PCM), and Toray Medical Co. Ltd. (Tokyo, Japan) (Polymethylmethacrylate-PMMA), were compared with Cuprophan® (Enka Ag, Wuppertal-Barmen, FRG) a cellulose-based membrane manufactured by the cuprammonium process, which is the most widely used haemodialysis membrane.

Leucopenia on reuse was studied for disposable dialysers containing Cuprophan and AN 69S membranes. Cuprophan-containing haemodialysers were reused by two different techniques, the first a manual technique in which the dialyser was reverse-flushed using reverse-osmosis treated water at the termination of dialysis. The second technique, which was also used for AN 69S-containing haemodialysers, was by an automated reuse system, ABG-Semca 704S [14], in which the dialyser's blood compartment was rinsed by a 0.5% sodium hypochlorite solution for a fixed period of 12 min. During this rinsing process the flow was intermittently pulsed by activation of a solenoid valve in the circuit. The sodium hypochlorite rinse was followed by a second rinse by formalin, followed by a filling phase in which both the blood and dialysate compartments were filled with formalin (5%).

Preparation of the dialyser prior to subsequent use was the same in both groups and involved water washing of the dialysate pathway for a minimum of 1 h, by treated tapwater, at a constant flow rate. Completion of the rinse period was followed by connection to the proportionating system. The blood lines were connected and the blood circuit rinsed by 1 litre

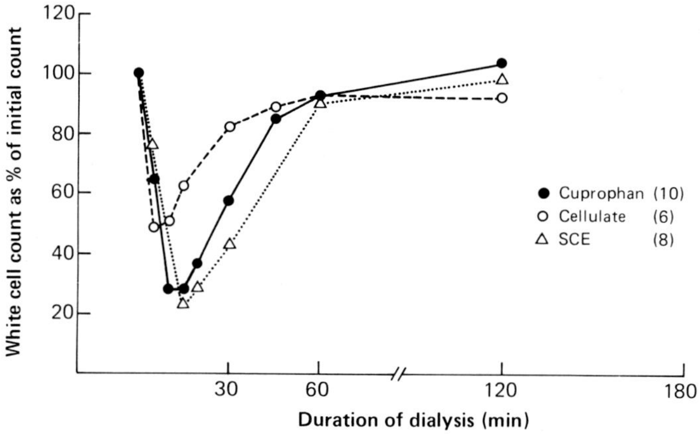

Fig. 1. Leucopenia observed with cellulose and modified cellulose haemodialysis membranes. Mean results shown. Figures in parentheses refer to number of studies.

of normal saline (0.9%). After 900ml had passed through the blood circuit, the saline effluent was tested for residual formalin by the use of Schiff's reagent. If the reaction was negative, the patient was connected to the extracorporeal circuit. Otherwise, a further rinse was undertaken.

Sampling

Predialysis blood samples were drawn from the arterial cannula at the time of insertion. Samples during treatment were drawn from the arterial segment of the extracorporeal circuit at 5, 10, 15, 20, 25, 30, 45, 60, 120 and 180min.

Heparin was used as an anticoagulant in all patients with an initial loading dose of 2,000IU injected into the arterial segment at commencement of dialysis followed by a continuous infusion of 1–2,000 IU/h, with the infusion being terminated at 45–60min prior to the end of dialysis. Blood samples were analysed on the same day using a Coulter counter.

Analysis of Results

All results have been expressed as a percentage of the initial or predialysis value to eliminate variations due to differences between patients' white cell counts. The statistical significance of the results was assessed by the analysis of variance.

Results

Effect of Different Membranes

Leucopenia for Cuprophan and modified cellulose membranes is shown in figure 1. In patients using Cuprophan, the mean (±SEM) white

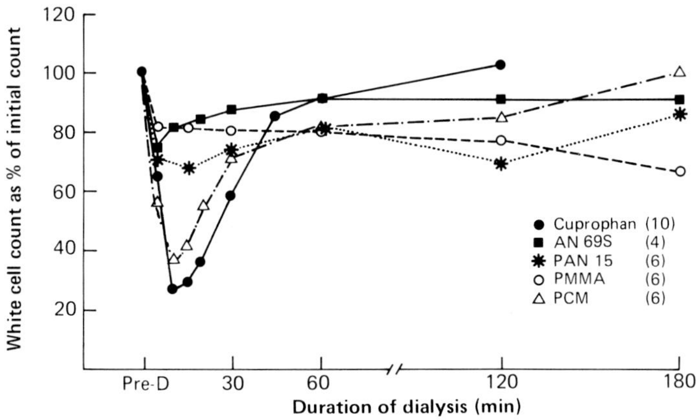

Fig. 2. Leucopenia observed with synthetic haemodialysis membranes. Mean results shown. Figures in parentheses refer to number of studies.

cell count at 15 min had fallen significantly and was 26.9 ± 3.6 % of the predialysis value. By 30 min it had risen (49.8 ± 3.9 %) and it continued to rise reaching predialysis levels by the second hour of dialysis. Patients using SCE showed comparable changes at 15 (23.4 ± 1.0 %) and 30 min (42.4 ± 2.9 %) and, in common with Cuprophan, predialysis levels were reached during the second hour of treatment.

Cellulate demonstrated a diminished response with white cell counts at 15 min of 63.1 ± 6.3 % while at 30 min, the mean had risen to 82.7 ± 2.9 % of the predialysis value.

A statistical comparison of these results failed to differentiate between Cuprophan and SCE. Differences between Cuprophan and Cellulate were significant at both 15 and 30 min ($p < 0.005$).

Leucopenia observed for the synthetic membranes studied is shown in figure 2. While cell count at 15 min for the Biospal 2400S haemodialyser containing AN 69S membrane was 82 ± 5.3 % of the predialysis value, and by 30 min it had risen marginally (88 ± 4.5 %) and remained at a comparable level throughout the remainder of dialysis. Haemodialysers containing PMMA and PAN 15 membranes demonstrated comparable changes. Polycarbonate demonstrated a more marked response with the white cell count at 15 min falling to 42 ± 3.3 % of the predialysis value. In common with the cellulose membranes, the mean value at 30 min had risen (72 ± 2.8 %) and predialysis values were achieved during the second hour of treatment.

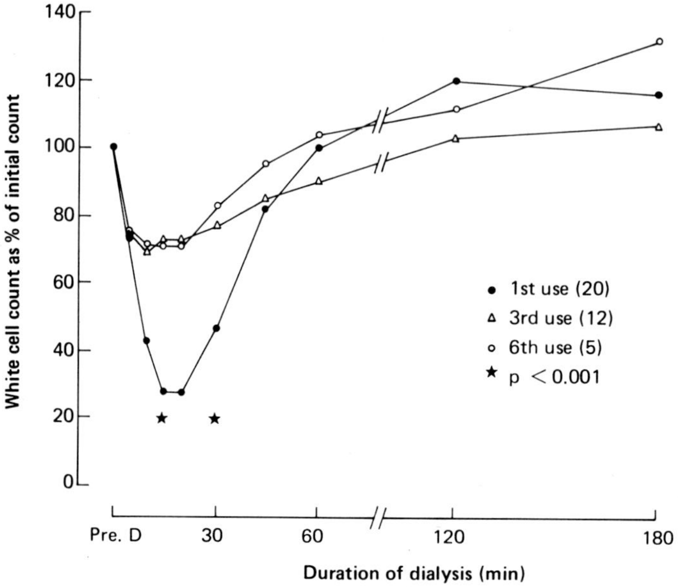

Fig. 3. Leucopenia observed in haemodialysers containing cellulose membranes (Cuprophan) after reverse osmosis water wash at the termination of dialysis. Mean results shown. Figures in parentheses refer to number of studies.

Statistically, no differences between synthetic membranes and Cuprophan could be demonstrated at 60min, but at 15 and 30min the differences between the two groups was highly significant; $p<0.001$ for AN 69S, PAN 15 and PMMA and $p<0.02$ for polycarbonate.

Changed Response after Reuse

Reuse of disposable and non-disposable dialysers is undertaken extensively in the United Kingdom [19] and the practice is growing elsewhere [7, 19]. White cell changes observed for Cuprophan containing haemodialysers reused without chemical rinsing (RO water wash) are shown in figure 3. By the third use (second reuse) the mean white cell count had risen to $72.5 \pm 3.6\%$ at 15min and was comparable at 30min ($77 \pm 3.7\%$). White cell changes during the sixth use of the dialyser (fifth reuse) were similar ($72.6 \pm 4\%$ at 15min, 83.3 ± 3.5 at 30min). Equivalent results for Cuprophan-containing dialysers rinsed with sodium hypochlorite showed no differences compared to first use (fig. 4). Chemical rinsing of AN 69S confirms this finding (table I).

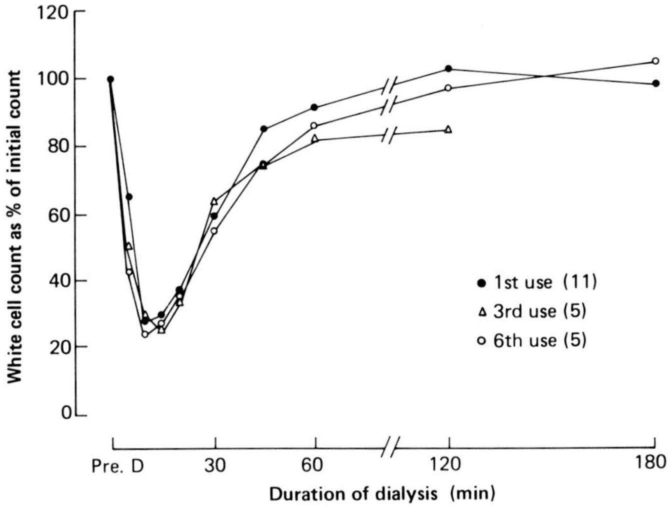

Fig. 4. Leucopenia observed in haemodialysers containing cellulose membranes (Cuprophan) after 0.5% sodium hypochlorite wash at the termination of dialysis. Mean results shown. Figures in parentheses refer to number of studies.

Table I. Haemodialysis leucopenia: influence of sodium hypochlorite on reuse of AN 69S membrane

	Use number		
Duration of dialysis, min	1	3	6
Pre-dialysis	100	100	100
+ 15	82 ± 3.9[1]	82 ± 4.6	83 ± 4.3
+ 30	88 ± 4.5	89 ± 5.1	90 ± 3.8
+ 45	91 ± 5.6	89 ± 2.7	91 ± 2.7
+ 60	91 ± 4.8	89 ± 2.0	91 ± 1.2
+120	90 ± 3.1	91 ± 5.5	89 ± 1.4
+180	90 ± 2.0	89 ± 3.9	91 ± 1.4
Number of dialysers studied	4	4	3

[1]White cell counts expressed as mean ± SEM % of predialysis value.

Discussion

The results obtained in the course of these studies confirm published findings [10, 12, 17] and demonstrate that cellulose membranes produce a more marked leucopenia than their synthetic counterparts. In the case of cellulose-based membranes our study shows that the chemical derivative of cellulose influences the magnitude of the changes. In the synthetic group of membranes studied AN 69S, PAN 15 and PMMA demonstrate comparable changes whereas polycarbonate is intermediate in its response. These differences may be related to the manufacturing process, the surface change of the membrane and its affinity for water.

The changed response as a result of reuse is well recognized [9, 11, 15, 18]. The explanation favoured by most authors is that during use a protective protein coating is laid down on the membrane. This protein coating is removed to a variable extent during the rinsing process at the termination of dialysis. Our studies demonstrate that improvements in biocompatibility may be observed but these improvements are a function of the treatment the membrane undergoes at the termination of dialysis. Exposure to hypochlorite, an agent used in a number of recently developed automated reuse systems negates any improvement possibly due to its action on the protein.

The clinical implications of these differences between cellulosic and noncellulosic membranes requires further study. Cellulose membranes have been in use for over 20 years and there are surviving patients who have received over 3,000 haemodialyses and have, presumably, been exposed to more than 3,000 episodes of leucopenia without apparent ill effects. In a previous study on small groups of patients, we demonstrated that the WBC count was higher in patients using polyacrylonitrile membranes than in patients using cellulose membranes [1]. However, this finding should be interpreted with considerable caution because at that time the polyacrylonitrile membrane could only be used with the recirculating system which was filled with dialysate manufactured using deionised water. Our cellulose membrane treated patients at the time were dialysed with fluid made from softened water, but it has since become apparent that softened water had a much higher aluminium content which led to chronic aluminium poisoning manifested by bone disease and in some cases, encephalopathy. It is now known that aluminium poisoning causes an irreversible macrocytic anaemia [16], so it is conceivable that it also affects the white cell count. At the moment, there is still a substantial cost difference between cellulose membranes and the synthetic alternatives and it would seem unreasonable to recommend a changeover on the basis of a laboratory phenomenon. Further comparisons of the comfort of dialysis and the long-term health of patients treated with cellulose and synthetic membranes in which all other variables eliminated as far as practicable, are clearly needed.

References

1 Aljama, P.; Conceicao, S.; Ward, M.K.; Feest, T.G.; Martin, A.M.; Craig, H.; Bird, P.A.E.; Sussman, M.; Kerr, D.N.S.: Comparison of three short dialysis schedules. Dialysis Transplant. *7*: 334–337 (1978).

2 Aurigemma, N.M.; Feldman, N.T.; Gottlieb, M.; Ingram, R.H., Jr.; Lazarus, J.M.; Lowrie, E.G.: Arterial oxygenation during hemodialysis. New Engl. J. Med. *297*: 871–873 (1977).

3 Burns, C.B.; Scheinhorn, D.J.: Hypoxemia during hemodialysis. Archs intern. Med. *142*: 1350–1352 (1982).

4 Brubaker, L.H.; Nolph, K.D.: Mechanisms of recovery from neutropenia induced by hemodialysis. Blood *38*: 623–631 (1971).

5 Craddock, P.R.; Fehr, J.; Brigham, K.L.; Kronenberg, R.S.; Jacob, H.S.: Complement and leukocyte mediated pulmonary dysfunction in hemodialysis. New Engl. J. Med. *296*: 769–774 (1977).

6 Craddock, P.R.; Fehr, J.; Dalmasso, A.P.; Brigham, K.L.; Jacob, H.S.: Hemodialysis leukopenia. Pulmonary vascular leukostasis resulting from complement activation by dialyzer cellophane membranes. J. clin. Invest. *59*: 879–888 (1977).

7 Deane, N.; Blagg, C.; Bower, J.; Palma, J. de; Gutch, C.; Kanter, A.; Ogden, D.; Sadler, J.; Siemsen, A.; Teehan, B.; Sosin, A.: A survey of dialyzer reuse practice in the United States. Dialysis Transplant. *7*: 1128–1130 (1978).

8 Graf, H.; Stummvoll, H.K.; Haber, P.; Kovarik, J.: Pathophysiology of dialysis related hypoxemia. Proc. Eur. Dial. Transplant Ass. *17*: 155–161 (1980).

9 Gral, T.; Schroth, P.; Palma, J.R. de; Maxwell, M.H.: Leukocyte dynamics during haemodialysis. Proc. Eur. Dial. Transplant Ass. *6*: 312–318 (1969).

10 Hakim, R.M.; Lowrie, E.G.: Hemodialysis-associated neutropenia and hypoxemia. The effect of dialyzer membrane materials. Nephron. *32*: 32–39 (1982).

11 Hakim, R.M.; Lowrie, E.G.: Effect of dialyzer reuse on leukopenia, hypoxemia and total hemolytic complement system. Trans. Am. Soc. artif. internal Organs *25*: 159–163 (1980).

12 Jacob, A.I.; Gavellas, G.; Zarco, R.; Perez, G.; Bourgoignie, J.J.: Leukopenia, hypoxia and complement function with different hemodialysis membranes. Kidney int. *18*: 505–509 (1980).

13 Kaplow, L.S.; Goffinet, J.A.: Profound neutropenia during the early phase of hemodialysis. J. Am. med. Ass. *208*: 133–135 (1968).

14 Man, N.K.; Glace, M.; Becker, A.; Di Giulio, S.; Zingraff, J.; Funck-Brentano, J.L.: A new dialyser re-use machine; in Frost, Conference on technical aspects of renal dialysis, 1977, pp. 73–79 (Pitman Medical, Tunbridge Wells 1978).
15 Savdie, E.; Bruce, L.; Vincent, P.C.: Modified neutropenic response to re-used dialyzers in patients with chronic renal failure. Clin. Nephrol. *8*: 422–428 (1977).
16 Short, A.I.K.; Winney, R.J.; Robson, J.S.: Reversible microcytic hypochromic anaemia in dialysis patients due to aluminium intoxication. Proc. Eur. Dial. Transplant Ass. *17*: 226–233 (1980).
17 Shin, J.; Matsuo, M.; Shinko, S.; Fujita, Y.; Inoue, S.; Sakai, R.; Nishioka, M.: A study on hemodialysis leukopenia using various dialyzers. J. Dial. *4*: 51–62 (1980).
18 Smith, E.K.M.; Jobbins, K.: Observations on neutropenia associated with haemodialysis. Br. med. J. *iv*: 70–73 (1969).
19 Wing, A.J.; Brunner, F.P.; Brynger, H.O.A.; Chantler, C.; Donckerwolcke, R.A.; Gurland, H.J.; Jacobs, C.; Selwood, N.H.: Mortality and morbidity of reusing dialysers. Br. med. J. *ii*: 853–855 (1978).

Dr. N.A. Hoenich, Department of Medicine, University of Newcastle upon Tyne, Newcastle upon Tyne, NE1 4LP (England)

Contr. Nephrol., vol. 37, pp. 129–133 (Karger, Basel 1984)

Haemodialysis Leucopenia as an Index of Membrane Biocompatibility

P. Aljama, J.M. Garin, A. Torres, A. Martin-Malo, E. Moreno, R. Perez-Calderon

Ciudad Sanitaria 'Reina Sofía', University of Cordoba, Spain

The appearance of selective neutropenia during haemodialysis was described by *Kaplow and Goffinet* [1] in 1968. This leucopenia occurs during the first 15–20min after the start of haemodialysis and is followed by a recovery of the number of neutrophils [1, 2]. *Craddock* et al. [3, 4] established that the leucopenia is a consequence of the activation of one or more components of the complement system caused by interaction between blood and the dialyser membrane. However, when polyacrylonitrile membrane dialysers are used no leucopenia is observed but the complement system becomes significantly activated [5]. In addition, *Henderson* et al. [6] using polysulfone membranes, observed no marked neutropenia but did demonstrate activation of complement. All this leads to the conclusion that the dialysis-induced leucopenia depends on the type of the dialyser membrane and is particularly related to conventional cuprophan haemodialysers. Moreover, it is tempting to speculate that complement activation is probably not the major responsible factor for dialysis neutropenia. These rapid changes in the number of peripheral neutrophils suggest that the leucopenia is due to the margination of neutrophils in the vascular bed. Indeed, *Craddock* et al. [7] demonstrated a significant increase in granulocyte margination, after the infusion of plasma exposed to cuprophan membranes. This experimental work also showed an entrapment of neutrophils in the pulmonary microcirculation as was previously demonstrated by *Toren* et al. [8].

These observations make the suggestion that the arterial hypoxemia and acute pulmonary dysfunction observed during the early phase of dialysis are mediated by the aggregation of granulocytes in the pulmonary vascular bed [7].

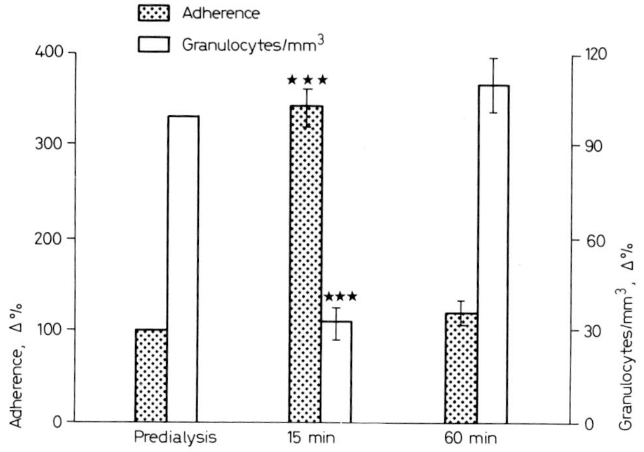

Fig. 1. Granulocyte adherence and count during dialysis with cuprophan membranes. ***$p<0.001$, paired t test.

Having presented all these facts, the overall clinical relevance of the neutropenia occurring during dialysis in respect to its short- and long-term consequences remains to be assessed. Furthermore, in view of the different neutrophil count behaviour with different types of membranes, this phenomenon might well reflect the degree of blood dialyser biocompatibility. For the last 2 years our group at the 'Reina Sofía' Hospital of the University of Cordoba has been interested in the study of the variations of granulocyte adherence during dialysis and its relationship to the leucopenia. We have also contemplated the role of the activation of the complement system and further hypothetic plasma factors involved in the mechanism of rapid-appearing neutropenia. Particular attention was paid to the granulocyte adherence changes because under experimental conditions in vitro adherence varies reciprocally with the peripheral leucocyte count [9].

We have modified the granulocyte adherence assay proposed by *MacGregor* [10, 11], using nylon fiber as surface for adherence. With cuprophan haemodialysers granulocyte adherence increases at the same time as the patients develop neutropenia. In fact, granulocyte adherence reaches the maximum at 15 min of dialysis which coincides with the time of granulocytopenia nadir. Both granulocyte count and adherence return to predialysis values at 60 min (fig. 1). These data show that cuprophan membranes induce augmentation of adherence and hence margination of the granulocytes, and the return to predialysis adherence value releases those

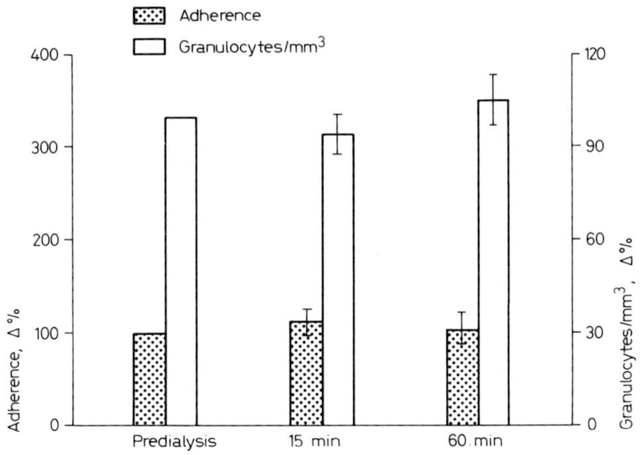

Fig. 2. Granulocyte adherence and count during dialysis with polyacrylonitrile AN-69 membranes.

white cells back to the peripheral circulating pool, recovering the granulocyte count at 60min of dialysis.

Figure 2 shows these findings in the same group of 10 patients during dialysis with polyacrylonitrile AN-69 membrane haemodialysers. As can be seen, there is no significant neutropenia nor any change in adherence during the period of the study. It appears therefore that when there is no increase in granulocyte adherence, neutropenia does not occur and both phenomena have a cause-effect relationship. *O'Flaherty* et al. [12] showed that in vivo complement activation increased granulocyte adhesiveness and circulating complement components are activated during cuprophan membrane haemodialysis [4]. From a series of relevant experiments, *Craddock* et al. [7] conclude that the adherence-augmenting factors, in patients being dialysed, are activated complement products. We have also studied the complement during dialysis and demonstrated that the same degree of activation is observed during cuprophan and polyacrylonitrile AN-69 membrane haemodialysis. In fact, figure 3 represents the levels of the total complement activity before and after 1h of dialysis with both types of membranes. As we reported [5, 13], once again, the same degree of activation of complement is induced with both types of membranes, despite the fact that significant neutropenia is absent during polyacrylonitrile haemodialysis.

Our findings strongly suggest that complement is not the major responsible factor for dialysis-induced leucopenia or that complement activa-

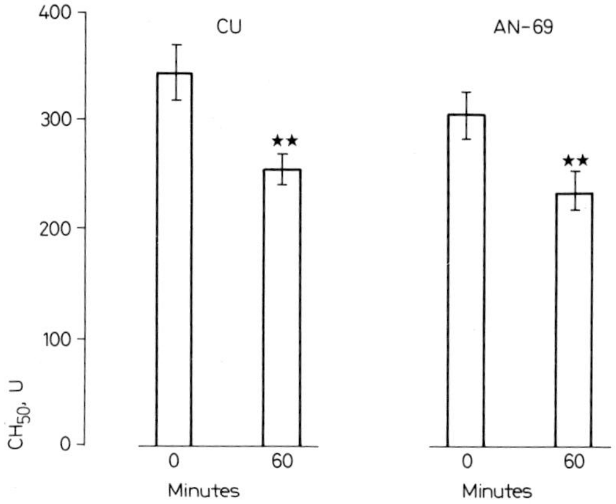

Fig. 3. Complement haemolytic activity changes during dialysis with cuprophan (CU) and polyacrylonitrile AN-69 membranes. $^{**}p<0.020$, paired t test.

tion may be the less important of two or more mechanisms of neutropenia. In this regard, *Woodward and Brubaker* [14] demonstrated that cuprophan-induced neutropenia is not prevented when the complement activation is inhibited by the administration of 5-hydroxyindoleacetic acid. At present it is sensible to propose that the degree of neutropenia observed during the early phase of haemodialysis reflects blood membrane biocompatibility. Complement activation seems, for the time being, inadequate to assess this important quality of any artificial membrane used in clinical extracorporeal circulation. Our data show the greater biocompatibility of the polyacrylonitrile AN-69 membrane dialysers, compared with the conventional cuprophan membranes. This could explain the better tolerance to the haemodialysis of a group of patients treated with these dialysers, particularly those suffering from cardiopulmonary dysfunction.

Model test systems are needed for the estimation of the membrane biocompatibility with screening purposes. It has recently been proposed that scanning electron microscopy in combination with microdensitometry are useful evaluating methods for blood compatibility of dialysers. However, in our hands, we have found these techniques unreproducible and in any case difficult to weigh up for large-scale comparative studies.

In summarizing, our studies to date show that the basic mechanism of haemodialysis-induced leucopenia is an increase in granulocyte adherence mediated by a plasma factor which seems independent of the complement system. Additionally, granulocyte adherence changes during dialysis may be considered as a reproducible index of membrane biocompatibility. Therefore polyacrylonitrile AN-69 membrane is shown to be superior, in this respect, to the conventional cuprophan biomaterials.

References

1 Kaplow, L.S.; Goffinet, J.A.: Profound neutropenia during the early phase of hemodialysis. J. Am. med. Ass. *203*: 1135–1137 (1968).

2 Gralt, T.; Schoroth, P.; De Palma, J.R.; Gordon, A.: Leucocyte dynamics with three types of hemodialysers. Trans. Am. Soc. artif. internal Organs *15*: 45–49 (1969).

3 Craddock, P.R.; Fehr, J.; Dalmaso, A.: Pulmonary capilary leukostasis: a complement (C) mediated complication of hemodialysis. Clin. Res. *23*: 402A (1975).

4 Craddock, P.R.; Fehr, J.; Dalmaso, A.P.; Brigham, K.L.; Jacob, H.S.: Pulmonary vascular leucostasis resulting from complement activation by dialyzer cellophane membranes. J. clin. Invest. *59*: 879–888 (1977).

5 Aljama, P.; Bird, P.A.E.; Ward, M.K.; Feest, T.G.; Walker, W.; Tanboga, H.; Sussman, M.; Kerr, D.N.S.: Haemodialysis induced leucopenia and activation of complement: effects of different membranes. Proc. Eur. Dial. Transplant Ass. *15*: 144–153 (1978).

6 Henderson, L.W.; Miller, M.E.; Hamilton, R.W.; Norman, M.E.: Hemodialysis leukopenia and polymorph random mobility: a possible correlation. J. Lab. clin. Med. *85*: 191–197 (1975).

7 Craddock, P.R.; Fehr, J.; Brigham, K.L.; Kronenberg, R.S.; Jacob, H.S.: Complement and leukocyte-mediated pulmonary dysfunction in hemodialysis. New Engl. J. Med. *296*: 769–774 (1977).

8 Toren, M.; Goffinet, J.A.; Kaplow, L.S.: Pulmonary bed sequestration of neutrophils during hemodialysis. Blood *36*: 337–340 (1970).

9 MacGregor, R.R.: Granulocyte adherence changes induced by hemodialysis, endotoxin, epinephrine and glucocorticoids. Ann. intern. Med. *86*: 35–39 (1977).

10 Guerrero, I.C.; Schreiber, A.D.; MacGregor, R.R.: Studies of the plasma factor which induces augmented granulocyte adherence during hemodialysis. Nephron *27*: 79–83 (1981).

11 MacGregor, R.R.; Spagnuolo, P.J.; Lentnek, A.L.: Inhibition of granulocyte adherence by ethanol, prednisone and aspirin, measured with a new assay system. New Engl. J. Med. *291*: 642–646 (1974).

12 O'Flaherty, J.T.; Craddock, P.R.; Jacob, J.S.: Effect of intravascular complement activation on granulocyte adhesiveness and distribution. Blood *51*: 731–739 (1978).

13 Aljama, P.; Conceicao, S.; Ward, M.K.; Feest, T.G.; Martin, H.; Graig, H.; Bird, P.A.E.; Sussman, M.; Kerr, D.N.S.: Comparation of three short dialysis schedules. Dialysis Transplant *7*: 334–337 (1978).

14 Woodward, J.; Brubaker, L.H.: Production of neutropenia-overshot cycle in sheep by reinfusion of cellophane exposed blood. Clin. Res. *21*: 56A (1973).

Dr. P. Aljama, Servicio de Nefrologia, Ciudad Sanitaria 'Reina Sofia', Córdoba (Spain)

Contr. Nephrol., vol. 37, pp. 134–141 (Karger, Basel 1984)

Hypoxemia during Hemodialysis: Effect of Different Membranes and Dialysate Compositions

W.A. De Backer[a], *G.A. Verpooten*[b], *D.J. Borgonjon*[a], *J.P. Van Waeleghem*[b], *P.A. Vermeire*[a], *M.E. De Broe*[b]

Departments of [a]Pneumology and [b]Nephrology-Hypertension, University of Antwerp, Belgium

Introduction

Kaplow and Goffinet [8] first reported the occurrence of a significant decrease in white blood cell (WBC) count, mainly granulocytes, between 2 and 15 min after the start of hemodialysis (HD). *Craddock* et al. [4, 5] suggested that this leucopenia was due to intrapulmonary leucostasis resulting from the activation of the alternative pathway of the complement system. These authors also found a decrease in arterial oxygen tension (PaO_2) soon after the start of HD and an increase in the calculated alveolo-arterial oxygen tension difference ($AaDO_2$). It was suggested that the parallel courses of the early leucopenia and hypoxemia soon after the start of HD were indicative of a causal relation between both phenomena.

Alternatively *Aurigemma* et al. [2] and *Dumler and Levin* [6] attributed the major cause of hypoxemia to alveolar hypoventilation subsequent to the loss of carbon dioxide (CO_2) in the dialysate. This was supported by their finding that no hypoxemia occurred if the decrease of PCO_2 in the dialysate was prevented. These results were only partially confirmed by *Tolchin* et al. [11], since in their 'constant PCO_2 dialysate set-up' they still found a small decrease in PaO_2. *Dolan* et al. [7] recently proposed once more that hypoventilation is the most important mechanism for the hypoxemia observed with acetate dialysis.

From a careful analysis of the studies mentioned above, it seems that the divergent conclusions could be explained partially by the use of different membranes known to induce different degrees of leucopenia.

The purpose of our study was to unravel the respective roles of the proposed mechanisms of HD-induced hypoxemia by performing four different HD combinations in 6 patients: two types of membranes with and without marked effects on blood leucocyte count and two types of dialysates with and without constant PCO_2. In two of these set-ups prostacyclin was also administered to evaluate further the role of leucocyte aggregation.

Methods

6 patients, aged 32–71 years, with terminal renal failure and treated by three weekly 4-hour HD sessions were studied. Their ventilatory function assessed by spirometry and body plethysmography was within normal limits. Vascular access consisted of an arteriovenous Cimino-Brescia type fistula. Heparin was administered under close control of anticoagulation.

Blood samples were drawn at 0, 15, 30, 60, 120, 180 and 240 min after the start of HD for blood gas measurements (pH, PO_2, PCO_2, HCO_3, BE) and WBC count. Expired gas was analyzed instantaneously using mass spectrometry in order to obtain alveolar oxygen tension (PAO_2). Alveolar carbon dioxide tension ($PACO_2$), mean expired oxygen tension (PEO_2) and mean expired carbon dioxide tension ($PECO_2$). $AaDO_2$ was calculated as the difference from end-tidal to PaO_2 measured simultaneously.

From recorded gas volumes (measured with a pneumotachograph) and the mixed expired gas concentration of oxygen and carbon dioxide, oxygen uptake ($\dot{V}O_2$) and carbon dioxide output ($\dot{V}CO_2$) were calculated as well as the respiratory quotient.

Differences from control values at time 0 were evaluated using Student's t test for paired observations.

Results

Effect of the Type of Membrane

Patients were studied during 4-hour acetate (AT) HD using different types of membranes. Cuprophane (CP) membranes (Gambro LP, 1 m^2-AB Gambro, Lund, Sweden) and polyacrylonitrile (PAN) membranes (Hospal 1 m^2, France) were used. The first membrane was chosen because of its well-known effect on blood leucocyte count, whereas the second has no such effect [1, 8]. If prostacyclin was used it was administered in a continuous infusion started 30 min before the start of HD at a dose of 8 ng/kg/min and continued during the whole HD procedure under close monitoring of the arterial blood pressure.

During HD using the CP membrane there was always an early decrease in PaO_2 (fig. 1), in HD using the PAN membrane changes in PaO_2

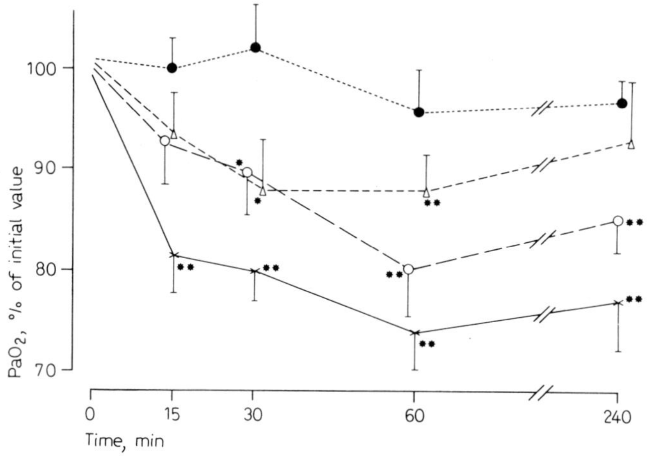

Fig. 1. Arterial oxygen tension (PaO_2) during hemodialysis (mean ± SE; n = 6). × = CP-AT (100% = 12.53 kPa); ○ = PAN-AT (100% = 13.03 kPa); △ = CP-BC (100% = 13.65 kPa); • = PAN-BC (100% = 12.47 kPa). Significance versus time 0: * $p < 0.05$; ** $p < 0.01$. Reprinted with permission from Kidney int. *23*: 738–743 (1983).

clearly depended on other factors (dialysate composition) and they could be absent. During prostacyclin infusion PaO_2 remained unchanged in HD with CP (fig. 2). Changes in PAO_2 could be present or absent during HD with either type of membrane and were clearly independent of it (fig. 3).

$AaDO_2$ always increased within the first hour using the CP membrane and remained unchanged using the PAN membrane (fig. 4). With prostacyclin $AaDO_2$ was also unchanged in CP-HD.

The increase in $AaDO_2$ consequent to ventilation-perfusion disturbances ($\dot{V}/Q$) clearly depended on the type of the membrane. In this respect measurement of $AaDO_2$ proved to be useful in evaluating the direct effect of the membrane on pulmonary gas exchange. WBC count rapidly decreased to 30% of control in the first 15 min of HD using CP but remained constant while using the PAN membrane. At the end of a 4-hour session WBC count was again within normal limits (fig. 5). Using prostacyclin the decrease in WBC count was less pronounced (fig. 2).

Effect of the Type of Dialysate

Patients were evaluated in the same way as in the membrane study. HD was performed using AT and bicarbonate (BC) containing dialysate. The PCO_2 of the BC-containing dialysate was kept constant around

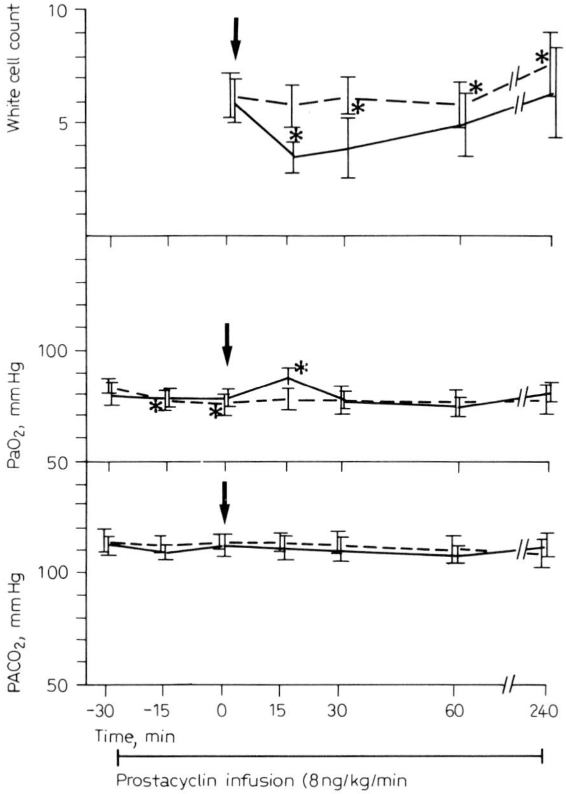

Fig. 2. Effects of prostacyclin infusion on white cell count, PaO_2 and $PACO_2$ before and during HD with cuprophan + bicarbonate (—) and PAN + bicarbonate (– – –). Means ± SE of 5 patients. ↓ = Start of hemodialysis. $^*p < 0.05$.

5.33 kPa using continuous mixing of two solutions[1] just before the dialysate reached the artificial kidney.

PaO_2 decreased more at the end of a 4-hour session during AT-HD than during BC-HD (fig. 1). PAO_2 always decreased during HD with AT (fig. 3). During HD with BC, alveolar hypoventilation was absent. Prostacyclin had no effect on PAO_2 during HD with BC (fig. 2). Changes in $AaDO_2$ were independent of the type of dialysate (fig. 4). They occurred as well during HD with AT as with BC. PCO_2 in the blood returning to the

[1] Solution 1: Na^+80 mEq/l; Ca^{++} 3.5 mEq/l; K^+ 1 mEq/l; Mg^{++}1 mEq/l; HCO_3^- 0 mEq/l; Cl^-85.5 mEq/l; Ac^-4 mEq/l. Solution 2: Na^+ 59 mEq/l; HCO_3^- 39 mEq/l; Cl^- 20 mEq/l.

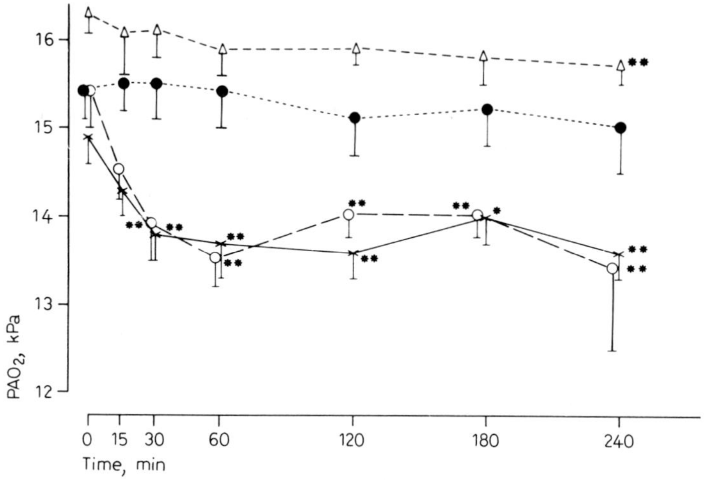

Fig. 3. Alveolar oxygen tension (PAO_2) during hemodialysis (mean ± SE; n = 6). × = CP-AT; ○ = PAN-AT; △ = CP-BC; ● = PAN-BC. Significance versus time 0: *p < 0.05; **p < 0.01. Reprinted with permission from Kidney int. *23*: 738–743 (1983).

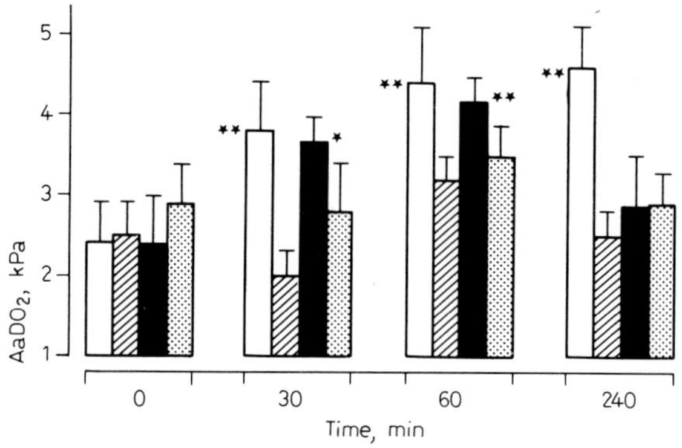

Fig. 4. Alveolar-arterial oxygen tension difference ($AaDO_2$) during hemodialysis (mean ± SE; n = 6). □ = CP-AT; ▨ = PAN-AT; ■ CP-BC; ▦ = PAN-BC. Significance versus time 0: *p < 0.05; **p < 0.01. Reprinted with permission from Kidney int. *23*: 738–743 (1983).

patient decreased to as low as 2 kPa (30% of normal value) in AT-HD, but remained constant in BC-HD. The decrease in the respiratory quotient reflects the decrease in the CO_2 content of the returning venous blood.

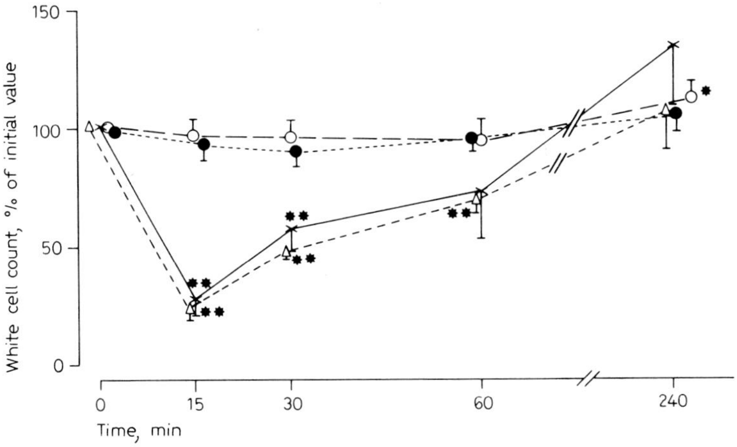

Fig. 5. White cell count during hemodialysis (mean ± SE; n = 6). × = CP-AT; ○ = PAN-AT; △ = CP-BC; ● = PAN-BC. Significance versus time 0: *$p<0.05$; **$p<0.01$. Reprinted with permission from Kidney int. *23*: 738–743 (1983).

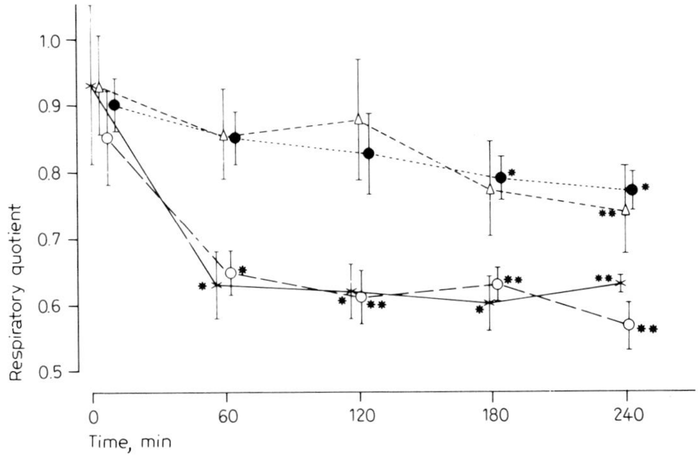

Fig. 6. Respiratory quotient during hemodialysis (mean ± SE; n = 6). × = CP-AT; ○ = PAN-AT; △ = CP-BC; ● = PAN-BC. Significance versus time 0: *$p<0.05$; **$p<0.01$. Reprinted with permission from Kidney int. *23*: 738–743 (1983).

Therefore in AT-HD a respiratory quotient as low as 0.55 could be observed, whereas the respiratory quotient was nearly unchanged in BC-HD (fig. 6).

Discussion

It appears from these results that the effect on arterial PO_2 and alveolo-arterial oxygen gradient is markedly different for CP and PAN membranes within minutes after the start of HD. Independent of the membrane, however, dialysate containing AT always induced a delayed but as striking decrease in PAO_2 and respiratory quotient. The use of a CP membrane is consistently associated with the rapid occurrence of an altered intrapulmonary gas exchange (increase in $AaDO_2$) and marked leucopenia.

The different effects on WBC counts suggest a better biocompatibility of the PAN membrane and it is quite tempting to speculate that the intrapulmonary changes are related to leucopenia. The role of leucopenia and leucocyte degranulations is questioned again in the experiments with prostacyclin in which less leucopenia and no early hypoxemia due to ventilation/perfusion disturbances occurs. Prostacyclin therefore could have presented leucocyte adhesion and degranulation as is well known from in vitro studies [3, 10]. Prostacyclin could also have influenced cardiac output with consequent changes in mixed venous and arterial PO_2.

The use of AT instead of BC in the dialysate was consistently associated with alveolar hypoventilation and hypoxemia. The latter could result from a direct effect of acetate by some as yet unclear mechanisms. Preliminary results from our group during hemofiltration with AC do not support this hypothesis. It seems more likely that the loss of carbon dioxide through the dialysate with PCO_2 in the blood returning to the patient decreasing to as low as 2 kPa causes alveolar hypoventilation and hypoxemia. *Phillipson* et al. [9] have recently demonstrated the critical dependence of respiratory drive and rhythmicity on the metabolic carbon dioxide overload by causing complete cessation of breathing at normal arterial blood gases in adult sheep when carbon dioxide was removed from the blood at a rate equal to its metabolic production.

In our patients we also found that hypoventilation occurs slowly and is not correlated with changes in arterial PCO_2. The suggestion that it could be mediated through slowly adapting chemoreceptors in the venous circulation or in the lungs, remains to be proven.

A decrease in PaO_2 of 25 %, as occurred in our study, e.g. in CP-HD, can be critical in patients with compromised cardiopulmonary functions and already low PaO_2 at the start of HD. The clinical implication of our results is clearly that those patients should preferentially be dialyzed with a biocompatible membrane and a dialysate in which loss of CO_2 is prevented.

Acknowledgement

We wish to thank Mr. *J. Geldhof* for technical assistance and Mrs. *A. Grootveld* for typing the manuscript.

References

1 Aliama, M.; Bird, P.A.E.; Ward, M.K.; Tanboga, H.; Sheridan, T.; Craig, H.; Kerr, D.N.S.: Hemodialysis-induced leucopenia and activation of complement: effects of different membranes. Proc. Eur. Dial. Transplant Ass. *15*: 144–153 (1978).

2 Aurigemma, N.M.; Feldman, N.T.; Gottlieb, M.; Ingram, R.H., Jr.; Lazarus, J.M.; Lowrie, E.G.: Arterial oxygenation during hemodialysis. New Engl. J. Med. *297*: 871–873 (1977).

3 Boxer, L.A.; Allen, J.M.; Schmidt, M.; Joder, M.; Bahner, R.L.: Inhibition of polymorphonuclear leucocytes adherence by prostacyclin. J. Lab. clin. Med. *95*: 672–678 (1980).

4 Craddock, P.R.; Fehr, J.; Brigham, K.L.; Kronenberg, R.; Jacob, H.S.: Complement and leucocyte mediated pulmonary dysfunction in hemodialysis. New Engl. J. Med. *299*: 769–774 (1977).

5 Craddock, P.R.; Fehr, J.; Dalmasso, A.P.; Brigham, K.L.; Jacobs, H.J.: Hemodialysis leukopenia: pulmonary vascular leukostasis resulting from complement activation by dialyzer cellophane membranes. J. clin. Invest. *297*: 879–888 (1977).

6 Dumler, F.; Levin, N.W.: Leucopenia and hypoxemia, unrelated effects of hemodialysis. Archs intern. Med. *139*: 1103–1106 (1979).

7 Dolan, M.J.; Whipp, B.J.; Davidsons, W.D.; Weitzman, R.E.; Wasserman, K.: Hypopnea associated with acetate dialysis: carbon dioxide-flow dependent ventilation. New Engl. J. Med. *305*: 72–75 (1981).

8 Kaplow, L.S.; Goffinet, J.A.: Profound neutropenia during the early phase of hemodialysis. J. Am. med. Ass. *203*: 1135–1137 (1968).

9 Phillipson, E.A.; Duffin, J.; Cooper, J.D.: Critical dependence of respiratory rhythmicity on metabolic CO_2 load. J. appl. Physiol. *50*: 45–54 (1981).

10 Rinaldo, J.E.; Rogers, R.M.: Adult respiratory-distress syndrome. Changing concepts of lung injury and repair. New Engl. J. Med. *306*: 900–909 (1982).

11 Tolchin, N.; Roberts, J.L.; Lewis, E.J.: Respiratory gas exchange by high efficiency hemodialyzers. Nephron *21*: 137–145 (1978).

M.E. De Broe, MD, Deparment of Nephrology-Hypertension, University Hospital, University of Antwerp, Wilrijkstraat 10, B–2520 Edegem (Belgium)

Contr. Nephrol., vol. 37, pp. 142–148 (Karger, Basel 1984)

Leukopenia and Complement Activation Induced by Different Dialysis Membranes

N.K. Man, N.Q. Tien, P. Lesavre, J.-L. Funck-Brentano[1]

Necker Hospital, Department of Nephrology, Inserm U-25 and U-90, University René-Descartes, Paris, France

Conventional dialysis membranes induce a transient marked leukopenia and activate complement [1–3]. This aspect of a noncellulosic membrane (polyacrylonitrile AN-69) and a new cellulosic membrane (cellulose acetate) were evaluated and compared to the Cuprophan membrane.

Material and Methods

Hematologic Studies

9 stable dialyzed patients were treated with an acetate-containing dialysate sequentially on three types of dialysis membranes: Cuprophan Enka (CU), cellulose acetate Cordis Dow (CA) and polyacrylonitrile Rhône-Poulenc (AN-69). Blood samples were withdrawn from the 'arterial' line for blood cell count and for differential white cell count at the start and at 10, 30 and 120 min of dialysis sessions. The results are expressed as percentage of predialysis levels (mean value of start samples) and the overall results for each membrane as the mean ± SEM. A paired t test was used to assess statistical significance.

Complement Activation Studies

In vitro. Calibrated membrane samples (1 cm^2 of each membrane cut into small pieces) were incubated in 100 μl of normal human serum (NHS) at 37 °C during 30 min. Complement activation was evaluated by the measurement of C_3 conversion rate by bidimensional immunodiffusion according to the *Laurell* [4] method. For the second phase of the immunodiffusion procedure, agarose plates were prepared with addition of 0.5 % anti-C3 serum in the

[1] We are indebted to *M.-H. Gaillard* and *D. Pierrat* for their technical assistance, to Hospal and Cordis Dow for their support.

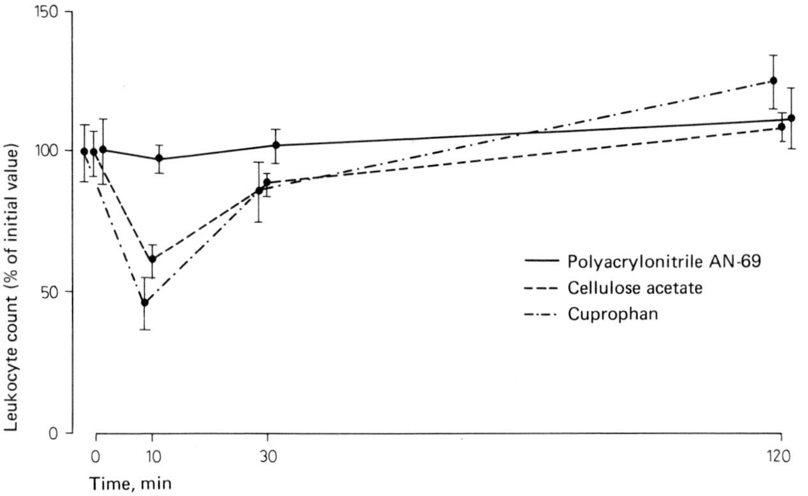

Fig. 1. Change in leukocyte count (% of initial value, Mean ± SEM) during 120 min of hemodialysis with three membranes: CU = Cuprophan; CA = cellulose acetate; AN-69 = polyacrylonitrile.

electrophoresis buffer. The results are expressed in percent of the ratio between the height of the C_3-converted bow and the total height of the two bows. Factor B-depleted serum and addition of Mg-EGTA to normal human serum were used to determine the complement activation pathway. Heparin was added to NHS in various amounts in order to study its inhibitory effect on complement activation induced by dialysis membranes.

In vivo. C3 cleavage was measured in blood samples withdrawn from the 'arterial' line at the start and at 10, 15, 30, 60, 120, 180, 240 and 300 min of a dialysis session from 3 patients treated on CU, CA and AN-69 membranes.

Results

Dialysis-Induced Leukopenia

Figure 1 shows the changes in leukocyte count during dialysis sessions performed with Cuprophan, cellulose acetate and polyacrylonitrile AN-69 membranes. At 10 min after the start, there was a marked leukopenia with Cuprophan: 45.7 ± 8.6 % of the initial value ($p < 0.001$, paired) and a less dramatic leukopenia with cellulose acetate: 60.9 ± 6.1 % of the initial value ($p < 0.001$, paried). The changes were minimal and not statistically significant with polyacrylonitrile AN-69. After 2 h of dialysis, rebound

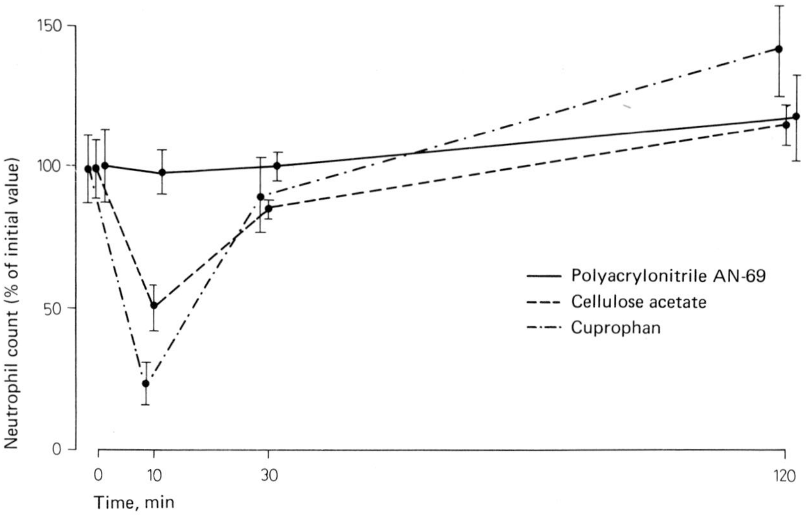

Fig. 2. Change in neutrophil count (% of initial value, mean ± SEM) during 120min of hemodialysis with three membranes.

leukocytosis was found for all the three membranes but was statistically significant ($p<0.001$, paired) only for the Cuprophan membrane. This transient leukopenia was mainly limited to neutrophils where the changes were similar (fig. 2). The thrombocyte count did not change significantly during hemodialysis run for all the three membranes.

Dialysis Membrane-Induced Complement Activation

In vitro Studies. Figure 3 illustrates the results obtained on agarose plates after electrophoresis in bidimensional immunodiffusion with NHS alone, NHS incubated with CU, and with AN-69 membrane. Reaction of the cellulose acetate membrane was similar to that of the Cuprophan membrane. The complement activation induced by cellulosic membranes was inhibited when EDTA was previously added in the incubation medium. When membrane samples were incubated with factor B-depleted serum, C_3 cleavage was less than 1%. On the contrary, addition of Mg-EGTA to normal human serum did not alter complement activation: 27 vs 24% when compared to normal human serum alone. The magnitude of complement activation by cellulosic membranes is surface area dependent. In our studies, about 12% C_3 cleavage per cm^2 per 100µl of NHS were found.

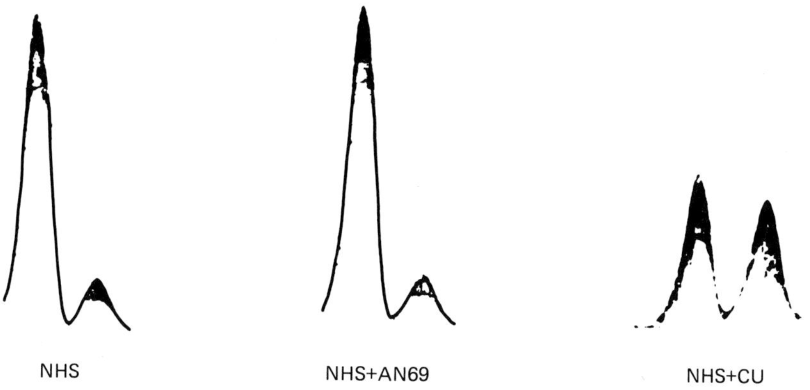

Fig. 3. In vitro complement activation induced by dialysis membranes. Precipitation pattern obtained when analyzing normal human serum with antigen-antibody crossed electrophoresis, using an anti-C_3 serum: normal human serum alone (NHS), incubated with polyacrylonitrile membrane (NHS + AN-69) and with cuprophan membrane (NHS + CU).

Heparin was inhibitory at 3–24 IU/ml: 3 IU/ml decrease complement activation by 50% and 24 IU/ml by 75%.

In vivo Studies. During a dialysis run made with cuprophan or with cellulose acetate membranes, maximum complement activation (10% C_3 cleavage) was found in the 15- and the 30-min plasma samples whereas complement activation was not detected in the 3-, the 4- and the 5-hour plasma samples. On the contrary, no complement activation was detected in any plasma samples from patients treated with the polyacrylonitrile AN-69 membrane.

Discussion

Cellulosic dialysis membranes are known to activate complement [3, 5]. No difference was noted between Cuprophan and other cellulosic membranes such as cellulose acetate. Activation of human complement induced by dialysis on cellulosic membranes is mainly through the alternative pathway, as demonstrated by the assays with factor-B depleted serum and with addition of Mg-EGTA to NHS. Only synthetic membranes such as polyacrylonitrile AN-60 or polycarbonate have no effect on human complement [5]. Our data on cellulosic dialysis membranes obtained by bidimensional immunodiffusion of C_3 conversion rate confirm the results of other groups using hemolytic titers of complement components as a functional measure of complement activity [3, 5, 6]. The measurement of C_3 cleavage by bidimensional immunodiffusion, used in this study, seems to be a more selective method and could explain the discrepancies found in assays made with polyacrylonitrile AN-69 membrane [5, 6]. Actually, these results could be predicted since cellulosic membranes are polysaccharide-based products which are capable of inducing complement activation [7].

From the early studies of *Ecker and Pillemer* [8] to the recent work of *Weiler* et al. [9], heparin has been known to possess anticomplementary as well anticoagulant activity. In the present study, heparin was inhibitory at 3–24 IU/ml. These concentrations are close to the levels obtained during therapeutic heparinization and could explain the differences between in vitro and in vivo studies on dialyzed patients.

The presence of C_3 degradation products in the arterial line of cellulosic membrane dialyzers has been demonstrated. The disappearance of this product within 2 h is probably due to high metabolic clearance and to an acquired inability to further activate the complement. This may be due to protein coating of the membrane [10]. A similar explanation could be presented for the lack of complement activation observed in reused cellulosic dialysis membranes [11].

The clinical implications of the transient complement activation found with cellulosic dialysis membranes are not well established. Continuous exposure to these membranes may potentially deplete complement proteins which in turn may predispose chronic hemodialysis patients to bacterial infections. However, *Jacob* et al. [6] found that there was no drop in titer of any complement component before dialysis and concluded that complement abnormalities are an unlikely explanation for the predisposition of dialysis patients to bacterial infections.

The relationship between exposure of plasma to cellulosic dialysis membranes and leukopenia is well established. However, the fall in leukocyte count in patients dialyzed against cellulose acetate membrane was less dramatic. This suggests that the chemical structure of membranes is involved in the generation of factors with potent effects on the physical properties of granulocytes [2, 12–14]. Complement activation during exposure of plasma to cellulosic dialysis membranes has been postulated to cause leukocyte-mediated hypoxia in hemodialysis patients. In spite of variable degrees of leukopenia, all the patients treated with an acetate-containing dialysate show, with any type of membrane, a similar and significant hypoxia, which was progressive throughout the dialysis run, even during the rebound leukocytosis phase [6]. The fact that hypoxia was also found in patients treated with a noncellulosic membrane, namely polyacrylonitrile AN-69 membrane [15], where neither leukopenia nor complement activation occurred, does not entirely support the mechanism presented by *Craddock* et al. [16]. Moreover, *Raja* et al. [17] demonstrated virtual elimination of hypoxia using bicarbonate-containing dialysate in patients treated with cellulosic membrane dialyzers.

It is more likely that hypoxia associated with acetate-containing dialysate results from loss of patient carbon dioxide and bicarbonate into the dialysate which ultimately depresses ventilation [18]. These data suggest that leukopenia and hypoxia may be concurrent but unrelated phenomena.

To what extent blood cell count changes and complement activation could be used as criteria for testing dialysis membrane biocompatibility remain questionable until clinical correlations are clearly established.

References

1 Kaplow, L.S.; Goffinet, J.A.: Profound neutropenia during the early phase of hemodialysis. J. Am. med. Ass. *203*: 133 (1968).
2 Gral, T.; Schroth, P.; Palma, J.R. de; Gordon, A.: Leukocyte dynamics with three types of hemodialysers. Trans. Am. Soc. artif. internal Organs *15*: 45 (1969).
3 Craddock, P.R.; Fehr, J.; Dalmasso, A.P.; Brigham, K.L.; Jacob, H.S.: Hemodialysis leukopenia. Pulmonary vascular leukostasis resulting from complement activation by dialyzer cellophane membrane. J. clin. Invest. *59*: 879 (1977).
4 Laurell, C.B.: Antigen-antibody crossed electrophoresis. Analyt. Biochem. *10*: 358 (1965).
5 Aljama, P.; Bird, P.A.E.; Ward, M.K.; Feest, T.G.; Walker, W.; Tanboga, H.; Sussman, M.; Kerr, D.N.S.: Haemodialysis-induced leucopenia and activation of complement. Effects of different membranes. Proc. Eur. Dial. Transplant Ass. *15*: 144 (1978).
6 Jacob, A.I.; Gavellas, G.; Zarco, R.; Perez, G.; Bourgoignie, J.J.: Leukopenia, hypoxia and complement function with different hemodialysis membranes. Kidney int. *18*: 505 (1980).
7 Muller-Eberhard, H.J.; Schreiber, R.D.: Molecular biology and chemistry of the alternative pathway of complement. Adv. Immunol. *29*: 1 (1981).
8 Ecker, E.E.; Pillemer, L.: Anticoagulant and complementary activity. An experimental study. J. Immun. *40*: 73 (1941).
9 Weiler, J.M.; Yurt, R.W.; Fearon, D.T.; Austen, K.F.: Modulation of the formation of the amplification convertase of complement C3bBb by native and commercial heparin. J. exp. Med. *147*: 409 (1978).
10 Vroman, L.; Klings, M.: Identification of proteins interacting at plasma-biomaterial interfaces. Proc. IXth Contractors' Conf. USDHEW, Bethesda, 1976, pp. 63.

11 Hakim, R.M.; Lowrie, E.G.: Effect of dialyzer reuse on leukopenia, hypoxemia and total hemolytic complement system. Trans. Am. Soc. artif. internal Organs *26*: 159 (1980).

12 Henderson, L.W.; Miller, M.E.; Hamilton, R.W.; Norman, M.E.: Hemodialysis leukopenia and polymorph random mobility. A possible correlation. J. Lab. clin. Med. *85*: 191 (1975).

13 Lentnek, A.L.; Schreiber, A.D.; McGregor, R.R.: The induction of augmented granulocyte adherence by Inflammation. Mediation by a plasma factor. J. clin. Invest. *57*: 109 (1976).

14 MacGregor, R.R.: Granulocyte adherence changes induced by hemodialysis, endotoxin, epinephrine and glucocorticoids. Am. intern. Med. *86*: 35 (1977).

15 Man, N.K.; Fournier, G.; Thireau, P.; Gaillard, J.L.; Funck-Brentano, J.-L.: Effect of bicarbonate-containing dialysate on chronic hemodialysis patients. A comparative study. Artif. Organs *6*: 421 (1982).

16 Craddock, P.R.; Hammerschmidt, D.; White, J.G., Dalmaso, A.P.; Jacob, H.S.: Hemodialysis leukopenia. Pulmonary vascular leukostasis resulting from complement activation by dialyzer cellophane membranes. J. clin. Invest. *59*: 879 (1977).

17 Raja, R.M.; Kramer, M.S.; Rosenbaum, J.L.; Bolisay, C.G.; Krug, M.J.: Hemodialysis associated hypoxemia. Role of acetate and pH in etiology. Trans. Am. Soc. artif. internal Organs *27*: 180 (1981).

18 Sherlock, J.; Ledwith, J.; Letteri, J.: Hypoventilation and hypoxemia during hemodialysis. Reflex response to removal of CO_2 across the dialyzer. Trans. Am. Soc. artif. internal Organs *23*: 406 (1977).

N.K. Man, MD, Hôpital Necker, Département de Néphrologie, 161, Rue de Sèvres, F-75015 Paris (France)

Contr. Nephrol., vol. 37, pp. 149–156 (Karger, Basel 1984)

Pregnancy in Patients with Pre-Existing Glomerular Disease

J.S. Cameron, J. Hicks
Renal Unit, Guy's Hospital, London, UK

The effect of pre-existing renal abnormality on the outcome of renal disease itself, and of the pregnancy, was examined in several series during the 1960s [1, 2]. It was already evident that hypertension was the major problem; the fetal loss rose fivefold [2] in the presence of hypertension, from 10 to about 50%. However, advances in safe hypotensive therapy during pregnancy, better fetal and maternal monitoring, and the advent of dialysis may have rendered these accounts obsolete. This paper reviews recent papers, and our own personal experience of 96 pregnancies, in 42 women with pre-existing *glomerular* disease, since it has been evident for some time that these patients present more problems than those women with tubulointerstitial disease, or polycystic kidneys [2].

We know now that the kidneys themselves are not necessary for successful completion of pregnancy, although substitution by dialysis is needed [3a]. In Europe about 20 women maintained on regular dialysis have born live babies, including 1 patient in our own unit [3b]. In general, uremic patients are not fertile, and even if not amenorrheic have a failure of ovulation. Regular periods often return during dialysis treatment. However, before the need for dialysis even patients with a GFR less than 10–20 ml/min have carried babies successfully, either without dialysis [4, 23] or with dialysis during the last trimester in those with the lowest levels of function [reviewed in ref. 30]. Most of these women were normotensive, however.

Neither is the presence of a nephrotic syndrome of itself a contraindication to a successful pregnancy, although *Studd and Blainey* [5] pointed out in 1969 that the babies born of nephrotic mothers were small in proportion to the degree of depression in maternal plasma albumin. The edema of the nephrotic state may be inconvenient, but should *not* be treated aggressively with diuretics, since we know that the fetal prognosis in idiopathic hypertension of pregnancy (so-called 'toxemia') varies with the maternal plasma volume [6], which is usually normal in nephrotic patients, but is reduced by diuretic therapy.

Interestingly, the response of the diseased kidney to pregnancy is normal, whether the primary disorder is glomerular or tubulointerstitial [7]. That is to say, the GFR rises along with – or in excess of – a rise in renal plasma flow which accompanies a normal expansion in maternal plasma volume and retention of sodium and water. All this takes place in the pregnant patient with pre-existing renal disease, and reduced renal function, but at a lower level throughout [7]. An important practical point is that one should *expect* some fall in creatinine clearance and a rise in plasma creatinine post-partum, along with the usual rise of 10–15mm Hg in the diastolic blood pressure. Particularly in patients in whom there are no pre-pregnancy data on renal function this may be interpreted wrongly, as evidence of a post-partum 'decline' in renal function.

Table I gives the outcome of a number of pregnancies documented in the literature and our own experience [23] in patients with pre-existing glomerular disease. Many forms of glomerular disease are more common in males and have a peak incidence over the age of 40, so experience is not large. In *minimal change disease* with a nephrotic syndrome the prognosis is (as might be expected) good, with only on occasional fetal loss and a low incidence of complicating hypertension. However a number of the babies were small for dates, and several of the labours were premature. In minimal change it is worth noting that prior treatment with cyclophosphamide, in women who had a nephrotic syndrome in childhood or adolescence but are now in remission (the usual outcome), there is no evidence as yet of an increase in fetal anomalies [23]. The prognosis for patients treated only with corticosteroids in the past in excellent [8, 23]. Equally, prednisone may be continued throughout pregnancy without problems if the patient is a 'frequent relapser', although many doctors would prefer to stop the treatment and take a chance on a relapse during pregnancy.

In *mesangiocapillary glomerulonephritis* (MCGN), in contrast to minimal change disease, an evolution to renal failure occurs in over 80% of patients eventually, and hypertension and reduced renal function are common. Thus, the outcome for the fetus might be expected to be worse, and this is born out by a fetal loss of 25%. This disease illustrates also the point that not only must one consider the effect of the renal disease on the pregnancy, but also the effect of pregnancy on the renal disease. *Fairley* [9]

Table I. Pregnancy in patients with various forms of glomerulonephritis

Glomerular disease	Number of pregnancies	Number of women	Therapeutic abortion	Fetal loss: spontneous abertion	Fetal loss: stillbirth	Fetal loss: neonatal	Fetal loss: total n	Fetal loss: total %	Maternal outcome: death	Maternal outcome: GFR ↓ reversible	Maternal outcome: GFR ↓ irreversible	Maternal outcome: BP ↑	References
Minimal change	33	22	4	2	0	1	3	10	0	0	0	2	5, 7, 10, 22, 23
FSGS	39	28	1	7	1	4	12	15	0	2	3	10	7, 10, 22–24
MCGN	58	37	14	8	0	3	11	25	2	4	1	18	7, 9, 10, 23
Membranous	72	54	7	7	0	0	8	12	0	2	1	10	5, 7, 9, 10, 22, 23 25, 26
IgA	52	34	1	0	2	5	7	14	0	2	0	17	10, 22, 23, 27
'Focal' GN	27	13	0	0	2	2	4	14	0	1	0	6	7, 23
'Proliferative' GN[1]	45	34	0	1	2	0	3	7	0	4	2	23	5, 7, 22
SLE	345	218	41	68	17	3	88	29	7 (3.2 %)	24	17	?	11–16, 23, 28–30

FSGS = focal segmental glomerulosclerosis; MCGN = mesangiocapillary glomerulonephritis; IgA = IgA-associated glomerulonephrophaty; SLE = systemic lupus erythematosus with nephritis.
[1]See text for explanation.

observed deterioration in renal function in a patient whose repeat biopsy showed crescents, and altogether 4 patients showed a reversible deterioration in renal function during pregnancy; 18/44 completed pregnancies were hypertensive.

Membranous nephropathy appears to carry a better prognosis for renal function, and most pregnancies going to term with live babies. Again, one of *Fairley's* [9] patients showed deterioration with the appearance of crescents but this has not been others' experience. The incidence of hypertension was almost entirely in the older report of *Studd and Blainey* [5], and again this adverse early experience has not been found since. There are few data on *focal segmental glomerulosclerosis*, and the incidence of neonatal deaths (4/25) in the Milan series [10] remains unexplained. The Milan group again provide some of the data on *IgA nephropathy*, the main difference between this and *Fairley's* [9] series being the incidence of hypertension during pregnancy (32 against 73%). We have too few patients to make any statement on this point. Finally, there are quite a few data from patients with 'proliferative glomerulonephritis' [7] from series in which, because of the early date of the biopsy, no precise classification can be given. In this group, as in all the others with structural damage, there was no increase in fetal loss.

The data in table I are of course influenced heavily by which women chose, or were encouraged to become pregnant, and which permitted their pregnancies to go to term, or to spontaneous abortion. This will obviously have been influenced by the doctor's advice, the emotional need for the woman to have a family, and the availability of contraception and therapeutic abortion. Thus, table I represents the outcome of those *selected from amongst possible pregnancies* in women with pre-existing glomerular disease, and does *not* represent either an unselected set of data or the natural history of pregnancy in this situation.

Thus most of the patients listed in table I had normal or near normal renal function, representing this process of selection. Within the group of patients with structural damage to the glomeruli (FSGS, MCGN, membranous, IgA, focal and proliferative) only patients with a pattern of mesangiocapillary glomerulonephritis appear to show a markedly higher fetal loss than usual. It is difficult, because of the varied origins of the data, to say exactly what level of fetal loss might be taken as a baseline. In the Milan series [10] and the data of *Katz* et al. [7], abortions and stillbirths were more common in hypertensive pregnancies whilst neonatal deaths were equally distributed. Of 198 pregnancies in this group of patients with structural glomerular damage allowed to proceed, 84 were complicated by de novo or pre-existing hypertension (42%), whilst only 15 pregnancies (8%) showed a reversible, and 7 (3.5%) an irreversible decline in maternal renal function. We have observed an irreversible decline in only a single patient of 40 in this group, a women with Alport's syndrome and focal segmental glomerulosclerosis whose GFR before pregnancy was only 30ml/min, complicated by severe hypertension. The 3 women in the FSGS group reported by *Taylor* et al. [24] who suffered loss of function all had uncontrolled hypertension.

Systemic lupus nephritis is of particular interest to obstetricians because it affects particularly young women of child-bearing age. The reproductive performance of patients who went on to develop clinical lupus later has been explained by several groups, including ourselves, but most carefully by *Fraga* et al. [11]. Of a total of 344 pregnancies in 125 women *prior* to the development of lupus [11–15, 23], there was a loss of 78/303 babies (26%). Because of the very diverse geographical origins of these data, it is even more difficult to say by how much this exceeds expectations, but it is undoubtedly high. Fertility did *not* appear to be impaired [11]. If women with *evident* lupus are considered (table I), the fetal loss is very similar (26%). The alarming point amongst these 345 pregnancies in 218 women is the maternal deaths (3.4%) which certainly exceeds expectations; 2 were in Mexico, 2 in Singapore, 2 in Italy and 1 in the USA. In the analysis of the 213 pregnancies in which the effect on maternal renal function was assessed, 26 showed a reversible and 17 an irreversible decline in renal function. How much of this was the result of inadequate management of hypertension is not possible to derive, but we have never seen either in 27 pregnancies. A post-partum 'flave' can be avoided by temporary escalation in steroid dose. All series point to an increased incidence of problems in pregnancy in those women with clinically-active SLE at the beginning of the pregnancy; the data of *Hayslett and Lynn* [16] on their collected series are particularly useful here. In this study there was a correlation between fetal loss and both active SLE and reduced renal function, but *not* a nephrotic syndrome with normal function, or with the pattern of glomerular disease seen in the renal biopsy; perhaps because many biopsies had been taken years previously.

The babies of women with SLE suffer additional risks besides the usual ones of hypertension, prematurity or a nephrotic syndrome. First, the mothers may be taking corticosteroids, sometimes azathioprine and occasionally cyclophosphamide. Fears that these regimes would have a markedly teratogenic effect on the fetus have, fortunately, proved groundless [*Davidson*, this volume]. Second, antibody of IgG class is transported across the placenta and thus autoantibodies directed against a number of tissues may enter the fetus, so that a positive antinuclear factor or a raised DNA binding are common in cord blood [17]; the infant may have a lupus rash, and suffer thrombocytopenia or pericarditis [18]. This syndrome is almost always transient and of no clinical significance. However, the problem of congenital heart block (which carries an appreciable mortality) *is* of importance [19]. Mothers with SLE give birth to babies with this complication much more frequently than normal, and, conversely, mothers with babies having congenital heart block go on to develop lupus. The pathogenesis is unknown, but may arise from fetal exposure to antibodies directed against bundle antigens. This mechanism of transplacental antibody may of course account for some of the high fetal loss in lupus, even in those with inactive disease and normal renal function. *Bresnihan* et al. [20] have suggested a correlation between lymphocytoxic antibodies in the other and fetal loss, but this was not confirmed by *Lom-Orta* et al. [31]. In addition, *Abramowsky* et al. [21] reported a decidual arteriopathy of immune origin, even in successful pregnancies with apparently inactive disease.

In summary the prognosis for women with pre-existing glomerular disease is good provided that their function is relatively normal, hypertension is absent or controlled and (in the case of SLE) disease is inactive. Little harm should come to the mother with meticulous antenatal care, particular attention being paid to the control of blood pressure *at levels normal for pregnancy* without the use of diuretics. However, even careful fetal monitoring has not eliminated an excess fetal loss, which is particularly marked in mothers with SLE, in whom it is present even before the clinical onset of the disease, and may well have an immunological component. The most important point in practice is close regular collaboration between obstetrician and nephrologist, and concentration of cases in few centres so that experience can be accumulated.

References

1 Mackay, E.V.: Pregnancy and renal disease. A ten year survey. Aust. N.Z. J. Obstet. *3*: 21–34 (1963).

2 Felding, C.: Pregnancy following renal diseases. Clin. Obstet. Gynec. *11*: 579–593 (1969).

3a Wing, A.J.; Registration Committee of the European Dialysis and Transplant Association: Successful pregnancies in women treated by dialysis and kidney transplantation. Br. J. Obstet. Gynaec. *87*: 839–845 (1980).

3b Marwood, R.P.; Ogg, C.S.; Coltart, T.; Klopper, A.I.: Plasma oestrogens in a pregnancy associated with chronic haemodialysis. Br. J. Obstet. Gynaec. *84*: 613–617 (1977).

4 Coward, R.A.; Mallick, N.P.; Warrell, D.W.; Crimes, D.; Kirkpatrick, H.: Successful pregnancy in severe chronic renal failure not requiring dialysis. Br. med. J. *iii*: 840–841 (1980).

5 Studd, J.W.W.; Blainey, J.D.: Pregnancy and the nephrotic syndrome. Br. med. J. *i*: 276–280 (1969).

6 Arias, F.: Expansion of intravascular volume and fetal outcome in patients with chronic hypertension and pregnancy. Am. J. Obstet. Gynec. *123*: 610–616 (1975).

7 Katz, A.I.; Davison, J.M.; Hayslett, J.P.; Singson, E.; Lindheimer, M.D.: Pregnancy in women with kidney disease. Kidney int., suppl., pp. 192–206 (1980).

8 Makker, S.P.; Heymann, W.: Pregnancy in patients who have had the idiopathic nephrotic syndrome in childhood. J. Pediat. *81*: 1140–1144 (1972).

9 Fairley, K.F.: Hypertension and renal disease in pregnancy. Proc. 8th Int. Congr. Nephrol., Athens, pp. 440–444 (Karger, Basel 1981).

10 Surian, M.; Imbasciati, E.; Cosci, P.; Banti, G.; Barbiano di Belgiojoso, G.; Brancaccio, D.; Minetti, L.; Ponticelli, C.: Glomerular disease and pregnancy. A study of 123 pregnancies in patients with primary and secondary glomerular diseases (submitted for publication, 1983).

11 Fraga, A.; Mintz, G.; Orozco, J.; Orozco, J.H.: Sterility and fertility rate, fetal wastage and maternal mortality in systemic lupus erythematosus. J. Rheumatol. *1*: 293–298 (1974).

12 Feng, P.H.: Systemic lupus erythematosus. A physician's viewpoint. Ann. Acad. Singapore *4*: 180–185 (1975).

13 Grigor, R.R.; Sherrington, P.C.; Hughes, G.R.V.; Hawkins, D.F.: Outcome of pregnancy in systemic lupus erythematosus. Proc. R.Soc. Med. *70*: 99–100 (1977).

14 Tozman, E.C.S.; Urowitz, M.B.; Gladman, D.D.: Systemic lupus erythematosus and pregnancy. J. Rheumatol. *7*: 624–632 (1980).

15 Imbasciati, E.; Surian, M.; Bottino, S.; Cosci, P.; Colussi, G.; Ambruso, G.C.; Massa, E.; Minetti, L.; Pardi, G.; Ponticelli, C.: Lupus nephropathy and pregnancy. A study of 30 pregnancies in patients with systemic lupus erythematosus and nephritis (submitted for publication, 1983).

16 Hayslett, J.P.; Lynn, R.I.: Effect of pregnancy in patients with lupus nephropathy. Kidney int. *18*: 207–220 (1980).

17 Beck, J.S.; Oakley, C.L.; Rowel, N.R.: Transplacental passage of antinuclear antibody. Study of infants of mother with systemic lupus erythematosus. Archs Derm. *93*: 656–663 (1966).

18 Doshi, N.; Smith, B.; Klionsley, B.: Congenital pericarditis due to maternal lupus erythematosus. J. Pediat. *96*: 699–701 (1980).

19 Chameides, L.; Truex, R.C.; Vetter, V.; Rashkind, W.J.; Galioto, F.M.; Noonan, J.A.: Association of maternal systemic lupus erythematosus with congenital complete heart block. New Engl. J. Med. *297*: 1204–1207 (1977).

20 Bresnihan, B.; Grigor, R.R.; Oliver, M.S.; Lewkonia, R.M.; Hughes, G.R.V.; Lovins,

R.E.; Faulk, W.P.: Immunological mechanism for spontaneous abortion in systemic lupus erythematosus. Lancet *ii*: 1205–1207 (1977).

21 Abramowsky, C.R.; Vegas, M.E.; Swinehart, G.; Gyves, M.T.: Decidual vasculopathy of the placenta in lupus erythematosus. New Engl. J. Med. *307*: 668–672 (1980).

22 Klockars, M.; Saarikoski, S.; Ikonen, E.; Kühlback, B.: Pregnancy in patients with renal disease. Acta med. scand. *207*: 207–214 (1980).

23 Cameron, J.S.; Hicks, J.: Unpublished observations.

24 Taylor, J.; Novak, R.; Christiansen, R.; Sorensen, E.T.: Focal sclerosing glomerulopathy with adverse effects during pregnancy. Archs intern Med. *138*: 1695–1696 (1978).

25 Forland, M.; Spargo, B.H.: Clinicopathological correlations in idiopathic nephrotic syndrome with membranous nephropathy. Nephron *6*: 498–525 (1969).

25 Noel, L.K.; Zanetti, M.; Droz, D.; Barbanel, C.: Long-term prognosis of idiopathic membranous glomerulonephritis. Study of 116 untreated patients. Am. J. Med. *66*: 32–90 (1979).

27 Kincaid-Smith, P.; Whitworth, J.A.; Fairley, K.A.: Mesangial IgA nephropathy in pregnancy. Clin. exp. Hypertension *2*: 821–838 (1980).

28 Boelaert, J.; Morel-Maroger, L.; Méry, J.P.: Renal insufficiency in lupus nephritis; in Hamburger, Crosnier, Maxwell, Advances in nephrology, vol. 4, pp. 249–289 (Year Book Medical Publishers, Chicago 1974).

29 Bear, R.: Pregnancy and lupus nephritis. A detailed report of six cases with a review of the literature. Obstet. Gynec. N.Y. *47*: 715–718 (1976).

30 Barnett, E.V.; Danovitch, G.M.; Lieb, G.M.: The influence of pregnancy on the systemic (non-renal) manifestations of systemic lupus erythematosus; in Fine (moderator), Systemic lupus erythematosus in pregnancy. Ann. intern. Med. *94*: 667–677 (1981).

31 Lom-Orta, H.; Diaz-Jouanen, E.; Alarcón-Segovia, D.: Lymphocytotoxic antibodies during pregnancy in systemic lupus erythematosus (Letter). Lancet *i*: 1034 (1979).

Prof. J.S. Cameron, Clinical Science Laboratories, 17th Floor, Guy's Tower, Guy's Hospital, London SE1 9RT (England)

Contr. Nephrol., vol. 37, pp. 157–169 (Karger, Basel 1984)

Renal Diseases and Pregnancy: Maternal and Fetal Disposition of Drugs

Giorgio Pardi, Patrizia Bozzetti, Annamaria Marconi

First Department of Obstetrics and Gynaecology, Perinatal Unit, University of Milan, Milan, Italy

Introduction

It is not uncommon that pregnancy arises in women affected with renal diseases and it is equally possible that renal pathology complicates an initially physiological pregnancy. The frequency of renal diseases in pregnancy is reported in table I. Data come from an epidemiological survey [1] sponsored by the National Research Council in five Italian cities from 1973 to 1979. In these cases often therapy is needed and a strict cooperation between obstetricians and nephrologists is essential: both must know all the problems related to drug use in pregnancy. Furthermore, the obstetricians' and/or nephrologists' duty must be to show in a realistic way the risks related to pregnancy in women of childbearing age affected with a renal disease and, if necessary, to indicate suitable measures for reducing these risks, or to recommend the most suitable contraceptive method.

Drugs and Pregnancy: General Problems

Drug administration in pregnancy must consider some factors which considerably modify the kinetics of the drug used: ingestion, absorption, distribution, metabolism, protein binding, and excretion. The pharmacologist can consider every single factor; the clinician must consider the whole result, since some factors act in the opposite direction. As regards the ingestion, it is necessary to remember, in cases of chronic administration, that 20–30 % of pregnant women vomit more or less frequently, espe-

Table I. Renal diseases and pregnancy: dimensions of the problem (32, 749 pregnancies)

	n	%
With previous renal disease	498	1.25
With hypertension	1,952	6.00
With urinary tract infections	873	2.70

cially during the first trimester. The reduced motility of stomach and gut can modify absorption. The physiological changes induced by pregnancy (e.g. increased plasma volume and total body water, increased body fat) and the presence of the fetoplacental unit can modify distribution. The increase in both renal plasma flow and glomerular filtration rate can interfere with excretion.

In the same way it is necessary to know the fetal side effects for drugs that cross the placenta. Moreover, still starting but with large prospects, a therapy specifically addressed to the fetus may be considered. At last, we must remember that some drugs can induce modifications on biophysical or biochemical parameters used for evaluating fetal welfare (fetal heart rate, urinary estriol: see next chapter).

Drugs Commonly Used in Pregnant Women with Renal Diseases

Antibiotics

Ampicillin is one of the most commonly used antibiotics in pregnancy. Figure 1 shows the serum concentration time courses of ampicillin after intramuscular injection of 10mg/kg to 14 pregnant and 6 nonpregnant women: note that the serum concentration is lower in pregnant women. Furthermore, since a level of 5μg/ml has been considered the adequate therapeutic concentration, antibiotic efficacy should be related to both time and intensity of bacterial exposure to levels higher than this. If we measure the area under the curve over that level we find significantly higher values in the nonpregnant than in the pregnant women (table II). The higher body clearance of ampicillin (a water-soluble molecule) by pregnant women can be explained on the basis of the physiological changes mentioned before: plasma volume, body water compartments (both intracellu-

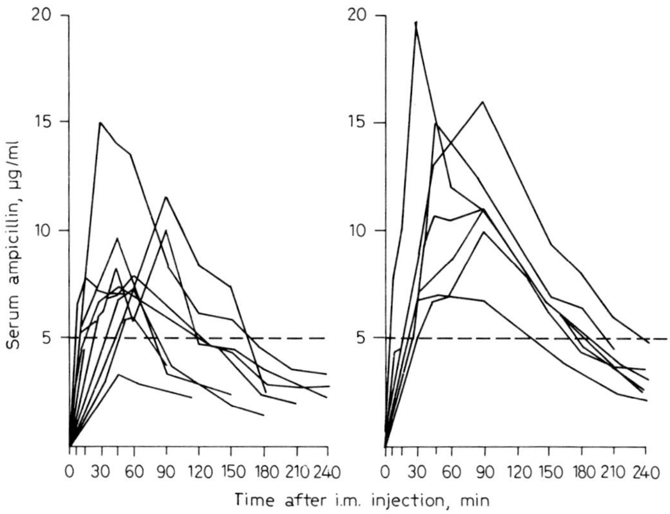

Fig. 1. Serum concentrations of ampicillin after intramuscular injection to pregnant (*a*) and nonpregnant (*b*) women. The mean values are indicated by the thick solid line. The dotted line indicates the adequate therapeutic ampicillin level.

Table II. Ampicillin after intramuscular injection (10 mg/kg)

	AUC µg ml^{-1} min		Body clearance ml^{-1}, min^{-1},kg
	total	5 µg/ml	
Nonpregnant	1,983 ± 649	675 ± 413	4.3 ± 1.2
Pregnant	1,243 ± 614*	209 ± 185**	7.7 ± 3.2*

AUC = Area under the serum concentration curve.
*$p<0.05$; **$p<0.01$.

lar and extracellular), renal blood flow increase as pregnancy advances. The higher volume of distribution will cause a lower serum concentration during pregnancy [2].

Studies performed by our group on the kinetics of gentamicin during pregnancy are reported in figure 2. Note that peak levels are reached at the same time in both groups, but in pregnant women serum concentration is lower. Apart from ampicillin and gentamicin a lower serum concentration during pregnancy has also been demonstrated for other antibiotics: cefazo-

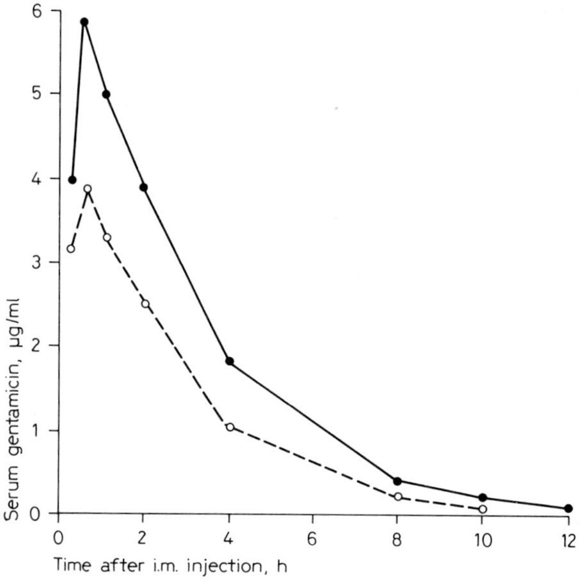

Fig. 2. Serum concentrations of gentamicin after intramuscular injection of 80 mg to pregnant (○) and nonpregnant (●) women.

lin, kanamycin, tobramycin. It can be concluded that for these drugs higher doses per kilogram body weight are required during pregnancy to reach adequate therapeutical levels and to avoid the risk of unsuccessful treatments. Furthermore, all these antibiotics reach the amniotic and fetal compartment [3]. As far as aminoglycosides are concerned, the potential risk of vestibular eight nerve damage must be considered with adequate postnatal follow-up.

Diuretics

The use of diuretic agents to treat hypertension and edema in pregnancy is still controversial as regards both efficacy and the benefit-to-risk ratio. These drugs do not seem to be useful in preeclampsia management, neither does their so-called prophylactic utilization seem to reduce the incidence of this disease [4].

Short courses of furosemide were included as an alternative diuretic in a randomized regional clinical trial to compare the efficacy of bed rest and pharmacological treatment. As very little is known about the disposition of furosemide in pregnancy, a pharmacokinetic protocol was included in the study [5]. Figure 3 shows the plasma concentration of furosemide at

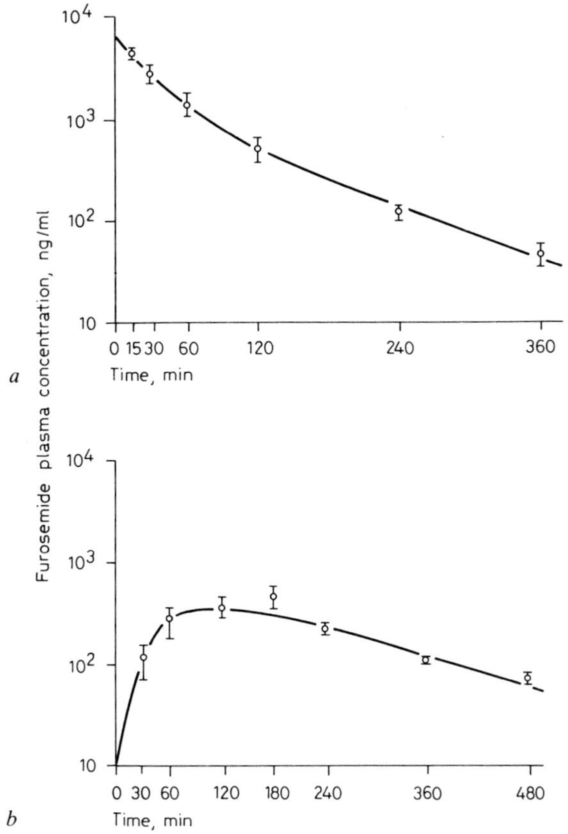

Fig. 3.a Furosemide plasma concentration (ng/ml) at various times after intravenous administration to 4 patients (mean ± SE). *b* Furosemide plasma concentration (ng/ml) at various times after oral administration to 8 patients (mean ± SE).

various times after intravenous (left) and oral (right) administration to 12 gestotic women: the maximum diuretic effect is reached during the first 2 h, after both intravenous and oral administration [5]. If we compare furosemide kinetics after intravenous injection in pregnant and nonpregnant women (table III), we can see that no differences are observed in elimination half-life time, volume of distribution, plasma clearance values and plasma protein binding [6, 7]. Furosemide crosses the placenta and levels measured in fetal blood shortly after administration to the mother equal those found in adults [6], (table IV). This specifically supports the finding that the drug has a pharmacological effect on fetal diuresis [8]. It must also

Table III. Furosemide kinetics after intravenous injection (40 mg)

	$t_{1/2}$, min	Total volume of distribution l/kg	Plasma clearance ml(min)	Plasma protein binding, %
Pregnant	71.8 ± 26.3	0.18 ± 0.02	152 ± 23	96 ± 1.3[a]
Nonpregnant[b]	71.8	0.181 ± 0.105	165.9 ± 42.4	96.3 ± 1.2

[a]Nonproteinuric women 96.6 ± 0.8, markedly proteinuric women 95.2 ± 3.2.
[b]From ref. 7.

Table IV. Maternal and cord plasma levels of furosemide

Case	Mother's levels ng/ml	Umbilical vein ng/ml	Umbilical artery ng/ml	Time after late administration, h
A	247	–	236	3.5
B	142	86.1 70.3	46.5 50.6	7.5

Patient B gave birth to twins.

be remembered that chronic treatment with diuretics increases the risk of fetal growth retardation [9].

Antihypertensives

This group of drugs is often used in pregnancy to treat mild and severe hypertension. On this subject it is necessary to know that in a high number of cases bed rest alone is effective. In a large study carried out in Lombardia [5] the hypertensive pregnant women (blood pressure ≥160/100) were divided into two groups, A and B, according to the presence or absence of edema. The protocol provided 3 days of bed rest before starting a pharmacological therapy. 36% of patients in group A and 47% in group B showed a persisting decrease in blood pressure values that allowed to avoid pharmacological therapy (fig. 4). On the whole, the kinetics of the antihypertensive drugs more commonly used in pregnancy is similar in both

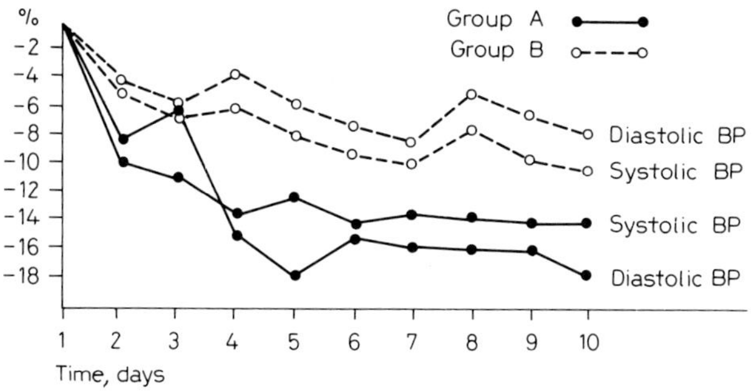

Fig. 4. Decrease of blood pressure after bed rest in hypertensive pregnant women (see also text).

pregnant and nonpregnant women: their molecular weight is generally low and hence they easily cross the placenta.

Reserpine, frequently used in the past years, is not recommended in pregnancy because it can decrease fetal catecholamine level and can induce Moro's syndrome in the newborn [10].

Alpha methyldopa is today commonly used in obstetric practice: the effectiveness of this drug in terms of reduction of maternal blood pressure and perinatal outcome is well documented by some controlled studies [4, 11]. However, a number of maternal and fetal side effects have been described. In the adult alpha methyldopa can induce toxic hepatitis [12], and in rabbit fetuses whose mothers received alpha methyldopa cardiac catecholamine levels were markedly reduced as compared to control fetuses [13]. This fact, due to transplacental passage of alpha methyldopa, could reduce fetal tolerance to hypoxia or other stress.

Hydralazine is also commonly used in obstetric practice. Many authors consider hydralazine as the first choice drug, intravenously for acute treatment of hypertensive crisis or orally for chronic treatment. Transplacental passage is documented in animals, however, specific fetal side effects related to hydralazine therapy have not been described in humans. Animal experiments have indicated that hydralazine may increase uteroplacental blood flow in sheep with hypertension [14].

Clonidine reduces blood pressure primarily by stimulating α-adrenergic receptor sites in the hypothalamus and other vasomotor centers in the central nervous system. It also suppresses the release of renal renin. It is not often used in pregnancy since many authors believe that other agents are preferable. However, in our Institute clonidine has been the first choice drug for a number of years. In our experience it appeared to be effective, with rare and unimportant maternal side effects. Chronic treatment with clonidine has been charged with inducing fetal bradycardia: in 88 hypertensive pregnant women treated by us with clonidine, fetal heart rate did not show any consistent change.

Controlled studies on the efficacy and maternal and fetal side effects of β-receptor blocking agents have been recently carried out [15] or are still in progress; therefore conclusive data are not yet available. It must be kept in mind that β-blockers cross the placenta and hence induce also a fetal β-blockade. In sheep fetuses, β-blockade reduces the tolerance to acute hypoxia. Risk of reduction of fetal heart rate must also be considered: maternal administration of propanolol has been proposed to obtain transplacental cardioversion in cases of fetal supraventricular tachycardia [16].

Corticosteroids

This group of drugs can be administered chronically in pregnant women with renal diseases (e.g. in systemic lupus erythematosus nephritis or after renal transplantation) and also, in acute conditions to prevent the respiratory distress syndrome of the neonate when premature delivery is foreseen. Transplacental passage of corticosteroids depends on placental metabolism: in vitro studies [17] have shown that placental inactivation of betamethasone and dexamethasone is negligible, while cortisol and prednisolone are largely inactivated (67% and 51%, respectively). The first two steroids are hence indicated when a fetal effect is desired while the last two are indicated when maternal therapeutical effects are needed. Transplacental passage of steroids induces depression of the fetal adrenal gland activity, as proved by the reduction of cortisol in cord blood after maternal administration of betamethasone. Inhibition is greatest after 7 days and lasts up to the 21st day [18]. Fetal adrenal gland production of estrogen precursor is also depressed and this is evidenced by reduction of plasma and urinary maternal estriol values [19] (fig. 5). Chronic administration of corticosteroids for maternal diseases increases the risk of cleft palate, but it is not charged with inducing other major malformations [20]; other adverse fetal effects (prematurity, growth retardation, death) may be attributed to the disease and not to the drug.

Azathioprine

This drug is currently used after renal transplantation to prevent rejection. In 1982 more than 1,000 pregnancies have been recorded in women

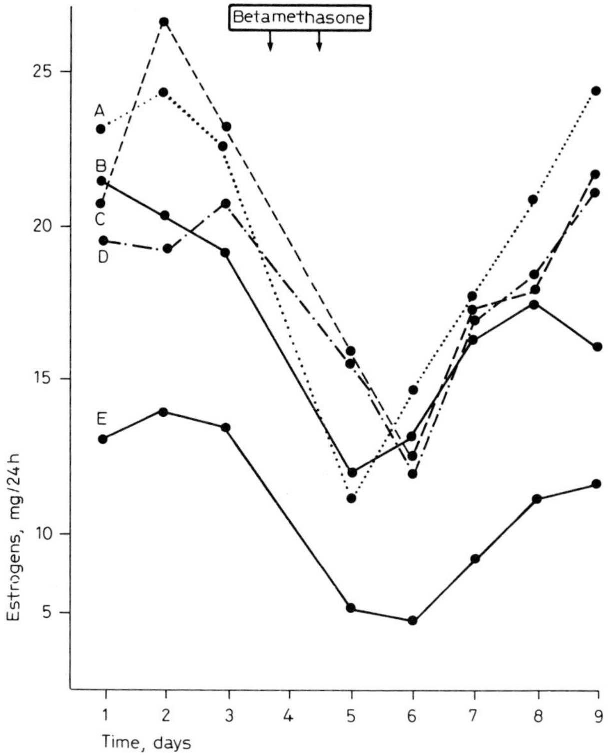

Fig. 5. Reduction of urinary estrogens after administration of 12 + 12 mg of betamethasone to the mother.

with previous renal transplantation. Experimental studies have shown that maternal administration of high doses of azathioprine in rats induces injuries to the blastocyst [21] and increases the risk of fetal growth retardation [22]. In the human, transplacental passage of azathioprine does not reduce fetal immunoglobulin synthesis [23]; however, the antimitotic effect of the drug certainly can be risk factor for fetal growth retardation [see the paper of *Davison* on pregnancy in renal transplant recipients, this volume]. In our Institute cytogenetic studies performed on fetal chromosomes in cases of chronic administration of azathioprine to the mother during pregnancy have shown a high frequency of chromosomal lesions (fig. 6; arrows indicate chromosomal fragmentation). These lesions were not accompanied by phenotypic alterations. For the future, when pregnancy is desired by a women with renal transplantation, reduction of azathioprine dosage may be considered.

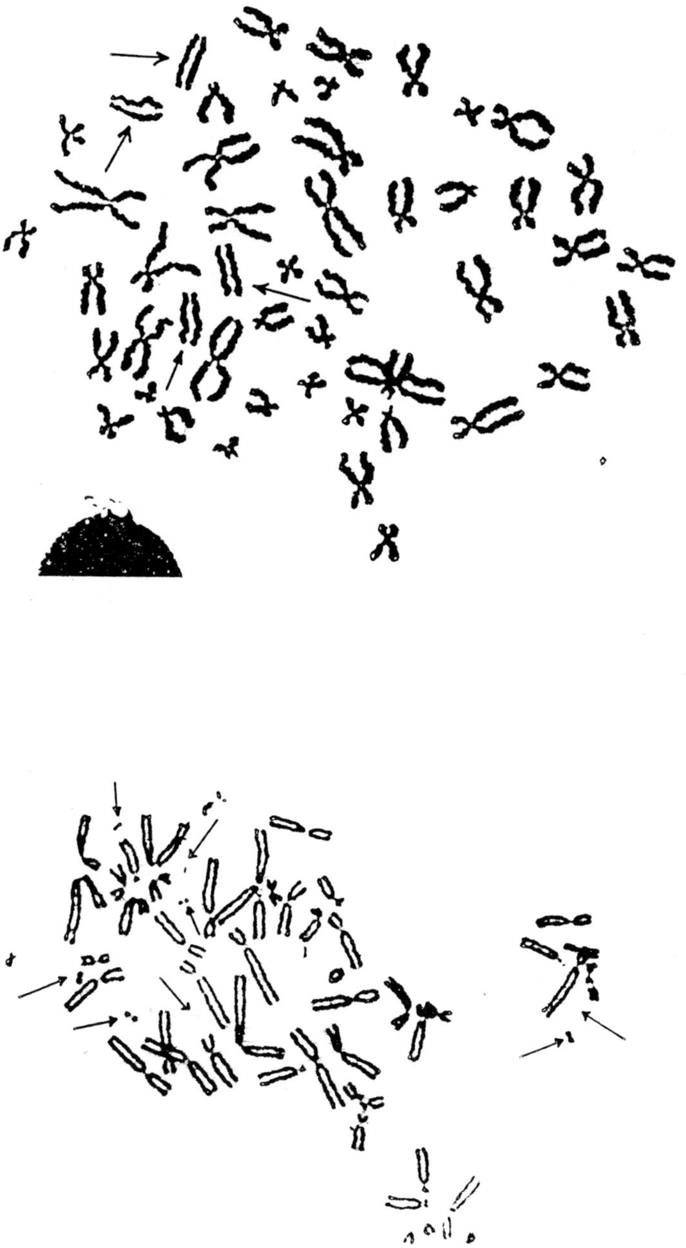

Fig. 6. Fetal chromosomal fragmentations (indicated by arrows) induced by chronic administration of azathioprine to the mother.

Conclusions

Renal diseases in pregnancy are not uncommon; many of them, preexisting or complicating pregnancy, require pharmacological therapy. In these cases strict cooperation between obstetricians and nephrologists is essential. During pregnancy, the kinetics of many drugs is modified due to changes in absorption, distribution, metabolism, excretion and protein binding. These changes are reflected in lower plasma concentration of some antibiotics such as ampicillin and aminoglycosides. Plasma concentrations and effects of other drugs (diuretics, antihypertensives) are similar both in pregnant and nonpregnant women. All these drugs easily cross the placenta and act on the fetus; transplacental passage and fetal side effects must be considered by the clinician, since they can interfere with fetal homeostasis and modify parameters commonly used for evaluation of fetal well-being.

Treatment of some renal diseases requires the use of corticosteroids and immunosuppressives: their administration should not be discontinued in pregnancy. Maternal consumption of corticosteroids induces depression of fetal adrenal gland activity, as demonstrated by lower cortisol levels in cord blood. Depression of the fetal adrenal gland is also proved by lower levels of estriol in maternal urine. Chronic treatment with corticosteroids is not charged with inducing major fetal malformations: unfavorable perinatal outcome (prematurity, fetal growth retardation or death) may be attributed to the disease more than to a direct effect of the drug on the fetus. A number of unfavorable fetal effects (chromosomal fragmentations, growth retardation) following transplacental passage of azathioprine have been described. For the future, when pregnancy is desired by a woman with renal transplantation, reduction of azathioprine dosage may be considered.

The risk-to-benefit ratio of pharmacological treatment in pregnant women with renal diseases is generally low: however, the factors related to the numerator must be carefully considered (and today are often underestimated) by good clinicians, both obstetricians and nephrologists.

References

1 Consiglio Nazionale delle Ricerche: L'indagine perinatale. Rapporto n° 2 (Pensiero scientifico, 1983).

2 Assael, B.; Como, L.; Miraglia, M.; Pardi, G.; Sereni, F.: Ampicillin kinetics in pregnancy. Br. J. clin. Pharmacol. *8*: 286 (1979).

3 Fisher, A.M.; Smith, M.R.: The prophylactic use of ampicillin and its transplacental passage after amniotomy. J. Obstet. Gynaec. Br. Commonw. *74*: 855 (1967).

4 Redman, C.W.G.: Treatment of hypertension in pregnancy. Kidney int. *18*: 267–278 (1980).

5 Pardi, G.; Barbato, M.; Bottino, S.; Tognoni, F.: Il trattamento dell'ipertensione in gravidanza: risultati di una ricera multicentrica in Lombardia. Annali Ostet. Ginec. Med. Perin. *102*: 391 (1981).

6 Riva, E.; Farina, P.; Tognoni, G.; Bottino, S.; Orrico, C.; Pardi, G.: Pharmacokinetics of furosemide in gestosis of pregnancy. Eur. J. clin. Pharmacol. *14*: 361 (1978).

7 Andreasen, F.; Mikkelsen, E.: Distribution, elimination and effect of furosemide in normal subjects and in patients with heart failure. Eur. J. clin. Pharmacol. *12*: 15 (1977).

8 Wladimiroff, J.W.: Effect of furosemide on fetal urine production. Br. J. Obstet. Gynaec. *82*: 221 (1975).

9 Campbell, D.; MacGillivray, I.: The effect of low caloric diet or a thiazide diuretic on the incidence of pre-eclampsia and on birth weight. Br. J. Obstet. Gynaec. *82*: 572 (1975).

10 Towell, M.E.; Hyman, A.I.; James, L.S.; Steinsland, O.S.; Gerst, E.C.; Adamsons, K.: Reserpine administration during pregnancy. Am. J. Obstet. Gynec. *92*: 711 (1965).

11 Redman, C.; Beilin, L.; Bonnar, J.: Treatment of hypertension in pregnancy with alpha methyldopa: blood pressure control and side effects. Br. J. Obstet. Gynaec. *419*: 426 (1977).

12 Rodman, J.S.; Deutsch, D.J.; Gutman, S.I.: Methyldopa hepatitis. Report of six cases and review of the literature. Am. J. Med. *60*: 941 (1976).

13 Hoskins, E.J.; Friedman, W.F.: Influence of maternal alpha methyldopa on sympathetic innervation in the newborn rabbit heart. Am. J. Obstet. Gynec. *137*: 496 (1980).

14 Brinkman, C.R.; Assali, N.S.: Uteroplacental haemodynamic response to antihypertensive drugs in hypertensive pregnant sheep; in Lindheimer, Katz, Zuspan, Hypertension in pregnancy, pp. 363–372 (Wiley, New York 1976).

15 Gallery, E.D.M.; Saunders, D.M.; Hunyor, S.N.; Gyory, A.Z.: Randomized comparison of methyldopa and oxprenolol for treatment of hypertension in pregnancy. Br. med. J. *1*: 1591 (1979).

16 Klein, A.M.; Holzman, I.R.; Austin, E.M.: Fetal tachycardia prior to the development of hydrops – attempted pharmacological cardioversion: case report. Am. J. Obstet. Gynec. *134*: 347 (1979).

17 Blanford, B.S.; Pearson Murphy, B.E.: In vitro metabolism of prednisolone, dexamethasone, betamethasone and cortisol by the human placenta. Am. J. Obstet. Gynec. *127*: 264 (1977).

18 Gennser, G.; Ohrlander, S.; et al.: Cortisol in amniotic fluid and cord blood in relation to prenatal betamethasone load and delivery. Am. J. Obstet. Gynec. *124*: 43 (1976).

19 Pardi, G.; Bottino, S.; et al.: La nostra esperienza nella prevenzione della sindrome respiratoria neonatale con corticosteroidi. Annali Ostet. Ginec. Med. Perin. *99*: 95 (1978).

20 Bongiovanni, A.M.; McPadden, A.: Steroids during pregnancy and possible fetal consequences. Fert. Steril. *11*: 181 (1960).

21 Gross, A.; Fein, A.; Serr, D.M.; Nebel, L.: The effect of Imuran on implantation and early embryonic development in rats. Obstet. Gynec. *50*: 713 (1977).

22 Scott, J.R.: Fetal growth retardation associated with maternal administration of immunosuppressive drugs. Am. J. Obstet. Gynec. *128*: 668 (1977).

23 Cederqvist, L.L.; Mercatz, I.R.; Litwin, S.D.: Fetal immunoglobulin synthesis following maternal immunosuppression. Am. J. Obstet. Gynec. *129*: 687 (1977).

G. Pardi, MD, First Department of Obstetrics and Gynaecology, Perinatal Unit, University of Milano, Via Commenda 12, I-20122 Milano (Italy)

Contr. Nephrol., vol. 37, pp. 170–178 (Karger, Basel 1984)

Pregnancy in Renal Transplant Recipients: Clinical Perspectives

J.M. Davison

MRC Human Reproduction Group, Princess Mary Maternity Hospital, Newcastle upon Tyne, UK

Chronic renal failure requiring dialysis is usually preceded by relative infertility and a variety of sexual disorders [1, 2]. Following transplantation there is rapid restoration of normal renal and endocrine function and it has been estimated that 1 of every 50 women of child-bearing age with a functioning renal transplant becomes pregnant [3]. Since 1970 there has been a marked increase in the number of pregnancies although analyses of any kind are likely to be underestimates as many must go unreported. Reviews have detailed the problems encountered [4, 5] and here the situation is brought up to date with a survey of 1,068 pregnancies in 717 patients.

The mean time between transplantation and conception was 40 months, with a range of 6 weeks to 13 years. 80% of the patients had received cadaver grafts, the exception being those in the series from Denver, USA (37 patients, 56 pregnancies) where 75% of the grafts had been donated by living relatives [6].

Early Pregnancy Outcome

28% of pregnancies ended in therapeutic abortion. Where given, the reasons included unplanned pregnancy, psychosocial problems, uncertainty about long-term maternal prognosis, unstable renal function before pregnancy, deteriorating renal function and/or severe hypertension in pregnancy and hereditary renal disease. Spontaneous abortion occurred in 13%, about the same as for the normal pregnant population. Thus 42% of all conceptions did not go beyond the first trimester, but of those that did, 90% ended successfully.

At least 0.5% of all conceptions were probably ectopic pregnancies. The diagnosis can be difficult because irregular bleeding and amenorrhoea may be associated with deteriorating renal function as well as an intra-uterine pregnancy [7]. A slightly higher risk of ectopic pregnancy must exist in transplant patients because of pelvic adhesions due to previous urological surgery or peritoneal dialysis, inflammatory disease or the overzealous use of intra-uterine contraceptive devices. The main clinical pitfall is erroneously attributing genuine gynaecological pathology to the transplant because of its location near the pelvis.

Course of Pregnancy

In the absence of severe maternal disease the hazards to the mother should be no more than those to which all renal transplant patients are subject. Nevertheless, there are problems but careful management usually ensures successful obstetric outcome. These patients must be monitored as high-risk cases, which requires attention to blood pressure, renal function, anaemia, infections of any sort and bone disease. Meticulous assessment of fetal growth is essential and is best performed by serial ultrasound assessment as urinary hormone excretion tests and probably plasma hormone levels are of no value [8]. Where there is evidence of severe intra-uterine growth retardation the possibility of congenital cytomegalovirus infection should be considered [9].

Allograft Function

The increase in glomerular filtration rate characteristic of early pregnancy is also evident in transplant recipients and the better the renal function before pregnancy the more satisfactory the obstetrical outcome [10]. There may be transient reduction in glomerular filtration rate during the third trimester just as occurs in normal pregnancy which does not represent a deteriorating situation with permanent impairment [11, 12]. Proteinuria occurs near term in about 40% of patients but disappears post-partum. Permanent impairment of renal function is occasionally seen especially where renal function is already compromised prior to conception [10, 13].

Pre-Eclampsia/Hypertension

Although the diagnosis of pre-eclampsia was made on clinical grounds in 30% of pregnancies this may not be a true picture. It is significant that biopsy studies in women with renal parenchymal disease have shown that the clinical diagnosis of superimposed pre-eclampsia can be wrong in about 50% of cases [14]. Furthermore, although many of the hypertensive syndromes occurring in renal transplant recipients are quite severe, there is only 1 report [15] of a woman (a primigravida) where there was rapid progress to eclampsia. Interestingly, she subsequently had a normal uncomplicated successful pregnancy [16].

From the management point of view serum uric acid levels and urinary protein excretion are not useful markers for either the onset or severity of pre-eclampsia in transplant recipients. Both indices can be substantially above the norm at any stage of gestation in otherwise uncomplicated pregnancies.

Allograft Rejection

Reports indicate that serious rejection occurs in 9% of women with pregnancies lasting into the third trimester [17]. While this incidence of rejection is no greater than expected for non-pregnant transplant patients, it could be considered unusual because the priviledged immunological state of pregnancy should benefit the transplant and there are reports of reduction or cessation of immunosuppressive therapy during pregnancy without rejection episodes [13, 18, 19]. Any effect of pregnancy seems to be unpredictable and is certainly not related to prior rejection episodes, the transplant-pregnancy time interval, problems in previous pregnancies or HLA types [20].

The diagnosis of rejection can be difficult but it should be suspected in the presence of certain clinical signs – fever, oliguria, hypertension and deteriorating renal function, often associated with renal enlargement and tenderness. Without biopsy confirmation, however, rejection cannot be distinguished from acute pyelonephritis, recurrent glomerulopathy and possibly severe pre-eclampsia [10]. The presence of pregnancy does not preclude the biopsy procedure, which should be undertaken before embarking upon anti-rejection therapy.

Infections

Most reports describe an increased incidence of all types of infection [13]. Patients should be carefully monitored for this possibility throughout pregnancy, particularly with regard to urinary tract infection and furthermore, prophylactic antibiotics should be given before any surgical procedure. The occurrence of viral infections in immunosuppressed patients is another potential hazard, both to mother and fetus [21].

Management of Delivery

Pre-Term Delivery (Delivery before 37 Weeks Gestation)

Pre-term delivery is common (50%) because of intervention for obstetrical reasons and the frequent occurrence of premature rupture of membranes or premature labour. Premature labour is also associated with poor renal function and this may be a contributory factor in some transplant patients [22]. In others, however, there is no obvious explanation, and it has been postulated that long-term steroid therapy may weaken connective tissues and contribute to the increased incidence of premature rupture of membranes [17].

Labour and Delivery

The transplanted kidney does not usually produce any mechanical dystocia during labour nor is it damaged during vaginal delivery. Although caesarian section is necessary for purely obstetrical reasons it is apparent from the literature that the incidence of 25% is more than might be anticipated. This presumably reflects fear of the unknown rather than a belief that vaginal delivery would damage mother and/or child.

Pelvic osteodystrophy may be a problem in these patients, related to their previous renal failure (and dialysis) or prolonged steroid therapy, particularly before puberty. Women with pelvic problems should ideally be recognised antenatally and delivered by caesarian section if there is cephalopelvic disproportion. Any doubts about the adequacy of the pelvis or kidney compression can be resolved by performing simultaneous urogram and X-ray pelvimetry at 36 weeks gestation [13]. Past history of pelvic infection or urological complications could imply difficulty in exposing the lower uterine segment [23] and occasionally a classical caesarian section may be necessary. Regardless of the route of delivery steroids must be augmented to cover the stress.

Paediatric Course

Neonatal Period

Over 50% of liveborns have no neonatal problems. There are no frequent or predominant developmental abnormalities. Pre-term delivery occurs in 50%, infants are small for gestational age in at least 20% and occasionally the two problems occur together. Immunogenetic disparity between a conceptus and its mother actually results in some apparent reproductive advantages, with placentae and fetuses being larger when greater maternofetal histoincompatibility exists. It is possible that non-specific depression of the immune system by an immunosuppressive agent like azathioprine could result in intra-uterine growth retardation [24], but the effect could also be explained by the direct cytotoxic action of azathioprine on the intra-uterine contents.

There are problems which are peculiar to the offspring of this group of patients. Thymic atrophy, transient leucopenia and thrombocytopenia, adrenocortical insufficiency, reduced blood levels of IgG and IgM, septicaemia, chromosome aberrations in lymphocytes, hypoglycaemia and hypocalcaemia have all been described [6, 13, 25–28].

Breast Feeding

A theoretical argument could be that as the baby has been exposed to azathioprine and its metabolites throughout pregnancy it should be well accustomed to them and that as their concentrations in breast milk are minimal then breast feeding is not contra-indicated [29]. Despite the beneficial effects of breast feeding, more specific information is needed about whether the amounts of azathioprine and its metabolites are trivial or substantial from a biological point of view [30, 31] and only then can sound advice be given.

Long-Term Course

Azathioprine can cause transient gaps and breaks in the chromosomes of lymphocytes [25–27]. Although they disappear spontaneously in 5–32 months, these anomalies may not be temporary in tissues not studied. The sequelae could be the eventual development of malignancies in the affected offspring or abnormalities in the next generation. It has been reported [32] that fertility problems affect the female offspring of mice that have been given low doses of 6-mercaptopurine, the main metabolite of azathioprine. These offspring subsequently prove to be sterile or, if they become pregnant, have smaller litters and more dead fetuses than do mothers that had not received the drug. Although there is reassuring information about general progress in infancy and early childhood [28, 33], there have been no studies on the possible impairment of fertility.

With the introduction of the new immunosuppressive agent cyclosporin A, which is supposedly more effective than conventional immunosuppression [34], new evaluations will be needed. To date, there is only one report of a pregnancy in a transplant patient taking cyclosporin A [35]. This pregnancy was non-complicated and the offspring's weight was appropriate for gestational age. As more data accrue an important question will be whether or not cyclosporin A is the agent of choice in transplant recipients contemplating pregnancy.

Children born to renal transplant mothers who are carriers of hepatitis B surface antigen probably become antigen carriers themselves [36, 37]. If the patient is an asymptomatic carrier the risk of the baby becoming antigen-positive is very low compared to 75 % in the presence of acute hepatitis in late pregnancy or within a few months after delivery [38]. There is usually little or no effect on general health but the baby's serum aminotransferases may be elevated perhaps signifying chronic persistent hepatitis, which in some cases has been verified by biopsy [37, 38]. The use of hyperimmunoglobulin against hepatitis B surface antigen given prophylactically to neonates has been investigated and it is known that the carrier state can be prevented in 75% if newborns are given hepatitis B immunoglobulin immediately after birth [39]. There can be little doubt that any child exposed to immunosuppression of any sort in utero should be under long-term surveillance.

Counselling Renal Transplant Patients

Until recently, the numerous case reports and registry data have focussed on the management of the pregnancy rather than the advisability of the initial conception. It is worrying that some pregnancies were not diagnosed until the second or third trimester, many patients believed that they could not conceive and 28 % of women requested or required termination of pregnancy. This situation must be tackled prospectively, contraceptive advice must be tailored to a particular patient's needs and pregnancy counselling must be offered to couples who want a child. All the long-term implications as well as those of pregnancy should be discussed. The medical establishment should not, however, adopt negative attitudes and if the situation is tackled prospectively patients rarely present the clinician with a fait accompli.

Pre-pregnancy assessment criteria have been published [4, 5, 40], but these are only guidelines and not strict rules. These are (a) good general health for 2 years after transplantation, (b) no proteinuria, (c) no significant hypertension, (d) no evidence of graft rejection, (e) no evidence of pelvicalyceal distension on a recent excretory urogram, (f) plasma creatinine of 180 μmol/l or less, and (g) drug therapy: prednisone, 15 mg/day or less, and azathioprine, 2 mg/kg/day or less.

Conclusions

All female transplant recipients of child-bearing age should be routinely advised about contraception, and couples who want a child should be encouraged to discuss all the implications. If a female recipient becomes pregnant, she must be monitored as a high-risk patient with her care involving the obstetrician, the nephrologists and eventually the paediatrician. In the absence of any severe maternal problems a successful obstetric outcome is usually achieved.

If further improvements in obstetric and neonatal care are to be achieved then emphasis should be placed on improving pre-pregnancy assessment criteria, studying the significance of hypertension and proteinuria, reassessing the rationale and implications of immunosuppression regimes during pregnancy, monitoring the effects of pregnancy on long-term renal prognosis and ensuring adequate follow-up of the offspring.

References

1 Lim, V.S.; Henriquez, C.; Sievertsen, G.; Frohman, L.A.; Ovarian function in chronic renal failure: evidence suggesting hypothalamic anovulation. Ann. intern. Med. *57*: 7–12 (1980).

2 Editorial: Effect of transplantation on non-renal effects of renal failure. Br. med. J. *284*: 221–222 (1982).

3 Editorial: Pregnancy after renal transplantation. Br. med. J. *i*: 733–734 (1976).

4 Davison, J.M.; Lindheimer, M.D.: Gynecologic and obstetrical problems after renal transplantation. Nieren-Hochdruckkrankheiten *11*: 258–265 (1982).

5 Davison, J.M.; Lindheimer, M.D.: Pregnancy in renal transplant recipients. J. reprod. Med. *27*: 613–621 (1982).

6 Penn, I.; Makowski, E.L.; Harris, R.: Parenthood following renal transplantation. Kidney int. *18*: 221–233 (1980).

7 Scott, J.R.; Cruikshank, D.; Corry, R.J.: Ectopic pregnancy in kidney transplant patients. Obstet. Gynec. *51*: 565–585 (1978).

8 Coulam, C.B.; Zincke, H.; Sterioff, S.: Pregnancy after renal transplantation: estrogen secretion. Transplantation *33*: 556–558 (1982).

9 Evans, T.J.; McCollum, J.P.K.; Valdimarsson, H.: Congenital cytomegalovirus infection after maternal renal transplantation. Lancet *i*: 1359–1360 (1975).

10 Davison, J.M.; Elliott, R.W.; Kerr, D.N.S.; Proud, G.; Taylor, R.M.R.; Ward, M.K.; Wilkinson, R.: Effect of pregnancy on renal function in kidney transplant recipients. Clin. exp. Hypertens. *B1*: 322 (1982).
11 Merkatz, I.R.; Schwartz, G.H.; David, D.S.; Stenzel, K.H.; Riggio, R.R.; Whitsell, J.C.: Resumption of female reproductive function following renal transplantation. J. Am. med. Ass. *216*: 1749–1754 (1971).
12 Rifle, G.; Traeger, J.: Pregnancy after renal transplantation: an international survey. Transplant. Proc. *7*: 723–728 (1975).
13 Sciarra, J.J.; Toledo-Pereyra, L.H.; Bendel, R.P.; Simmons, R.L.: Pregnancy following renal transplantation. Am. J. Obstet. Gynec. *123*: 411–425 (1975).
14 Katz, A.I.; Davison, J.M.; Hayslett, J.P.; Singson, E.; Lindheimer, M.D.: Pregnancy in women with kidney disease. Kidney int. *18*: 192–206 (1980).
15 Williams, P.F.; Jelen, J.: Eclampsia in a patient who had had a renal transplant. Br. med. J. *ii*: 972 (1979).
16 Williams, P.F.; Johnstone, M.: Normal pregnancy in renal transplant recipient with history of eclampsia and intrauterine death. Br. med. J. *285*: 1535 (1982).
17 Rudolph, J.E.; Shwihizir, R.T.; Barius, S.A.: Pregnancy in renal transplant patients: a review. Transplantation *27*: 26–29 (1979).
18 Kaufman, J.J.; Digman, W.; Goodwin, W.E.; Martin, D.C.; Goldman, R.; Maxwell, M.H.: Successful normal childbirth after kidney homotransplantation. J. Am. med. Ass. *200*: 162–165 (1967).
19 Davison, J.M.; Dellagrammatikas, H.; Parkin, J.M.: Fetal haematopoiesis and azathioprine therapy in pregnant patients with renal transplants. Clin. exp. Hypertens. *B1* 209 (1982).
20 Guttman, R.D.: Renal transplantation (I and II): New Engl. J. Med. *301*: 975–981, 1038–1048 (1979).
21 Spencer, E.S.; Anderson, H.K.: Viral infections in renal allograft recipients treated with long term immunosuppression. Br. med. J. *ii*: 829–830 (1979).
22 Felding, C.F.: Obstetric aspects in women with histories of renal disease. Acta obstet. gynec. scand. *48*: 2–43 (1969).
23 Editorial: Urological complications of renal transplantation. Br. med. J. *285*: 394–395 (1982).
24 Scott, J.R.: Fetal growth retardation associated with maternal administration of immunosuppressive drugs. Am. J. Obstet. Gynec. *128*: 441–444 (1971).
25 Leb, D.E.; Weisskopf, B.; Kanovitz, B.S.: Chromosome aberrations in the child of a kidney transplant recipient. Archs intern. Med. *128*: 441–444 (1971).
26 Lower, G.D.; Stevens, L.E.; Najarian, J.S.; Reemtsma, K.: Problems from immunosuppressive during pregnancy. Am. J. Obstet. Gynec. *111*: 1120–1121 (1971).
27 Price, H.V.; Salaman, J.R.; Laurence, K.M.; Langmain, H.: Immunosuppressive drugs and the fetus. Transplantation *21*: 294–298 (1976).
28 Korsch, B.M.; Klein, J.D.; Negrete, V.F.; Henderson, D.J.; Fine, R.N.: Physical and psychological follow-up on offspring of renal allograft recipients. Pediatrics *65*: 275–283 (1980).
29 Verco, C.J.; Hawkins, D.F.: Pregnancy after renal transplantation. J. Obstet. Gynaec. *3*: 29–33 (1982).
30 Fagerholm, M.I.; Coulam, C.B.; Moyer, T.P.: Breast feeding after renal transplantation: 6-mercaptopurine content of human breast milk. Surg. Forum *31*: 447–449 (1980).

31 Coulam, C.B.; Moyer, T.P.; Jiang, N.-S.; Zincke, H.: Breast-feeding after renal transplantation. Transplant. Proc. *14*: 605–609 (1982).
32 Reimers, T.J.; Sluss, P.M.: 6-Mercaptopurine treatment of pregnant mice: effects on second and third generations. Science *201*: 65–67 (1978).
33 Rasmussen, P.; Fasth, A.; Ahlmén, J.; Brynger, H.; Iwarson, S.; Kjellmer, I.: Children of female renal transplant recipients. Acta paediat. scand. *70*: 869–875 (1981).
34 European Multicentre Trial. Cyclosporin A as sole immunosuppressive agent in recipients of kidney allografts from cadaver donors. Preliminary results of a European multicentre trial. Lancet *ii*: 57–60 (1982).
35 Lewis, G.J.; Lamont, C.A.R.; Lee, H.A.; Slapak, M.: Successful pregnancy in a renal transplant recipient taking cyclosporin A. Br. med. J. *286*: 603 (1983).
36 Schweitzer, I.L.; Dunn, A.E.; Peters, R.L.; Spear, R.L.: Viral hepatitis B in neonates and infants. Am. J. med. *55*: 762–771 (1973).
37 Skinhöj, P.; Cohn, J.; Bradbourne, A.F.: Transmission of hepatitis type B from healthy HbsAg-positive mothers. Br. med. J. *i*: 10–11 (1976).
38 Dalquist, E.; Nordenfelt, E.: Neonatal hepatitis type B: a three year follow-up. Scand. J. infect. Dis. *6*: 305–308 (1974).
39 Recommendations of the Immunization Practices Advisory Committee: Immune globulins for protection against viral hepatitis. Ann. intern. Med. *96*: 193–197 (1982).
40 Davison, J.M.; Uldall, P.R.; Lind, T.: Planned pregnancy in a renal transplant recipient. Br. J. Obstet. Gynaec. *83*: 518–527 (1976).

J.M. Davison, MD, MRC Human Reproduction Group, Princess Mary Maternity Hospital, Newcastle upon Tyne, NE2 3BD (UK)

Contr. Nephrol., vol. 37, pp. 179–181 (Karger, Basel 1984)

Effects of Hypertension on Renal Function in Pregnant Rats

A. Dal Canton, M. Sabbatini, C. Esposito, M. Altomonte, G. Romano, F. Uccello, G. Conte, G. Fuiano, D. Russo, V.E. Andreucci

Department of Nephrology, Second Faculty of Medicine, University of Naples, Italy

Introduction

Recently, we have shown a marked fall in afferent arteriole resistance in pregnant rats [1]. This renal vasodilatation might blunt renal autoregulation in pregnancy, allowing for systemic hypertension to determine profound modifications in intrarenal hemodynamics, and hence in renal sodium handling. This study was performed to investigate the effects of hypertension on renal function in pregnant rats.

Methods

The studies were carried out in adult female Munich-Wistar rats, with glomeruli on the kidney surface, in which a silver clip (0.2mm i.d.) was placed on the right renal artery under light ether anesthesia. After this maneuver, in 8 rats systolic blood pressure (measured daily by the tail-cuff method) rose over 140mm Hg and remained elevated throughout the study. These were the hypertensive rats. In other 8 rats, instead, systolic blood pressure remained steadily normal (<140mm Hg) despite insertion of the clip. These were the normotensive controls. All the rats were fed on a standard chow containing 0.12mmol Na^+/g and, after placing the clip, received hypotonic saline (50mmol NaCl/l) to drink, instead of tap water. This policy of increasing Na^+ intake was necessary because in preliminary studies all of 10 rats with 2-kidney, 1-clip hypertension, receiving the standard Na^+ intake, became normotensive with pregnancy. After giving saline to drink, instead, only 15% of hypertensive rats had to be discarded from the study due to normalization of blood pressure during pregnancy.

Metabolic Studies

After placing the clip, all the rats were allowed to stabilize for 3 weeks, and then were mated for 2 days, the second of which was taken as day 1 of pregnancy. In the last 3 days before mating, and from the 2nd to the 14th day of pregnancy, the rats were housed in individual metabolic cages. During metabolic housing, sodium and water balance, body weight, and systolic blood pressure (tail-cuff) were monitored daily.

Micropuncture Studies

At the end of metabolic studies, the rats were anesthetized and the left kidney was exposed for renal micropuncture, as previously described [2]. Micropuncture measurements included all parameters of glomerular dynamics. Technical details and methods of calculation have been thoroughly described in our previous papers [1, 3, 4].

Results

Metabolic Studies

During pregnancy, systolic blood pressure ranged between 145 and 180mm Hg in hypertensive rats, and between 115 and 135mm Hg in normotensive controls. Body weight was similar in hypertensive as in control rats before mating (180.0 ± 7.1 vs. 183.7 ± 23.4g), but rose less during pregnancy in hypertensive rats (14th day: 200.0 ± 16.0vs. 211.8 ± 20.7g, $p<0.05$). Cumulative Na^+ excretion in days 3–14 of pregnancy averaged 48.4mmol in hypertensive rats, and 31.4mmol in controls ($p<0.01$). Cumulative Na^+ intake averaged 57.7mmol in hypertensive rats, and 45.1mmol in controls ($p<0.01$). Cumulative Na^+ balance (Na^+ retained) averaged 9.3mmol in hypertensive rats vs. 13.7mmol in controls ($p<0.05$). Similarly as for Na^+, hypertensive rats excreted more water than controls (301.7 vs. 141.8ml, as a mean), and introduced more water, too (mean 527.8 vs. 392.8ml). Cumulative water balance (water intake−water excretion) was lower in hypertensive than in normotensive rats (mean 226.1 vs. 251.0ml).

Micropuncture Studies

During micropuncture studies, mean blood pressure from femoral artery (systolic + ⅓ pulse pressure) averaged 124.5mm Hg in hypertensive rats vs. 98.0 in controls ($p<0.01$). Single nephron GFR (SNGFR) was moderately, but not significantly higher in hypertensive rats than in controls (mean 38.3 vs. 33.1ml/min); glomerular plasma flow (GPF) averaged 218.6nl/min in hypertensive rats and 110.1nl/min in controls ($p<0.05$), accounting for a lower single nephron filtration fraction (SNFF, mean 0.24 vs. 0.32) in hypertensive rats.

Discussion

In this study, hypertensive rats excreted more salt and water than normotensive controls in the first 2 weeks of pregnancy. This enhanced natriuresis and diuresis in hypertensive rats was only in part compensated for by a greater Na^+ and water intake; in hypertensive rats, in fact, cumulative retention of Na^+ and water during pregnancy was reduced, accounting for a lower increase in body weight. Micropuncture studies showed a higher glomerular plasma flow in hypertensive rats than in controls, indicating impaired renal autoregulation in the former. SNGFR, instead, was similar in the 2 groups and, therefore, SNFF was lower in hypertensive rats.

The lower SNFF may account, at least in part, for the greater Na^+ and water excretion in hypertensive rats, by reducing peritubular oncotic pressure and hence passive fluid reabsorption in the proximal tubule [5]. In addition, defective renal autoregulation may be responsible for natriuresis and diuresis, by allowing transmission of a higher hemodynamic pressure within vasa recta and, therefore, reducing Na^+ reabsorption in Henle's loop [6].

References

1 Dal Canton, A.; Conte, G.; Esposito, C.; Fuiano, G.; Guasco, R.; Russo, D.; Sabbatini, M.; Uccello, F.; Andreucci, V.E.: Effects of pregnancy on glomerular dynamics: micropuncture study in the rat. Kidney int. *22*: 608–612 (1982).

2 Andreucci, V.E.: Manual of renal micropuncture (Idelson, Naples 1980).

3 Dal Canton, A.; Stanziale, R.; Corradi, A.; Andreucci, V.E.; Migone, L.: Effects of acute ureteral obstruction on glomerular hemodynamics in rat kidney. Kidney int. *12*: 403–411 (1977).

4 Dal Canton, A.; Corradi, A.; Stanziale, R.; Maruccio, G.F.; Migone, L.: Effects of 24-hour unilateral ureteral obstruction on glomerular dynamics in rat kidney. Kidney int. *15*: 457–462 (1979).

5 Brenner, B.; Falchuk, K.; Keimowitz, R.; Berliner, R.: The relationship between peritubular capillary protein concentration and fluid reabsorption by the renal proximal tubule. J. clin. Invest. *48*: 1519–1531 (1969).

6 Dal Canton, A.; Conte, G.; Fuiano, G.; Guasco, R.; Andreucci, V.E.: Exaggerated natriuresis in the hypertensive man: a clinical evidence for intrarenal hemodynamic heterogeneity. Nephron *27*: 122–126 (1981).

A. Dal Canton, MD, Department of Nephrology, Second Faculty of Medicine, University of Naples, I-80100 Naples (Italy)

Contr. Nephrol., vol. 37, pp. 182–189 (Karger, Basel 1984)

Pregnancy and Course of Primary Glomerulonephritis

C. Rovati, M.L. Perrino, G. Barbiano di Belgiojoso, M. Surian, L. Radaelli, L. Minetti

Divisione di Nefrologia e Dialisi, Ospedale Niguarda Ca'Granda, Milano, Italia

Introduction

The effect of pregnancy on renal diseases is still unclear. Some investigators [1, 2] claim that gestation does not negatively influence the course of glomerulonephritides; by contrast, others reported a worsening of the glomerular lesions and a deterioration of renal function [3].

By a combined prospective and retrospective study, we analyzed the influence of pregnancy on renal function profile in patients with primary glomerulonephritis (GN).

Materials and Methods

Between 1970 and 1982, in the Nephrology and Obstetrics Departments of the Milano Ca'Granda Hospital, 29 patients with primary GN, who underwent 48 pregnancies after the diagnosis of kidney disease, were observed. The patients were distributed into the following classes according to the type of GN: class A, Berger's disease, 13 cases; class B, membranous glomerulonephritis (MGN), 3 cases; class C, focal segmental glomerulosclerosis (FSGS) 8 cases; class D, membranoproliferative glomerulonephritis (MPGN), 5 cases. Present nephrotic syndrome was observed in 0, 1, 3 and 2 cases, respectively, and early hypertension in 3, 2, 3 and 0 cases, respectively. These patients were compared with a control group of 23 GN patients matched as to the type of GN (11 Berger's disease, 3 MGN, 7 FSGS, 2 MPGN), mean age, duration of follow-up, renal function, proteinuria and blood pressure at the beginning of the observation.

Selective criteria for all groups were: normal renal function at the beginning of the study; histological diagnosis established by kidney biopsy (light microscopy, immunofluorescence, electronmicroscopy); at least one gestation to the third trimester. The control group included patients who were never pregnant or in whom any relation between the onset of renal disorder and previous gestation could be excluded. Secondary glomerulopathies were accurately excluded. The follow-up, limited for both groups to the child-bearing age, ranged from 12 months to 20 years. Whenever possible the length of follow-up was approximated yearly.

Renal function profile was drawn from serum creatinine concentrations at the beginning of the observation and at the end of the follow-up. The progression rate of GN was evaluated by linear regression analysis of the reciprocal of the serum creatinine concentration versus time [5]. This analysis was carried out both in gravidas (before and after pregnancy) and in the control group.

In the case of multiple pregnancies the period 'before' was considered before any gestation and the 'after' was initiated after the last one. The plasma creatinine measurement more approximated to the closest year was selected.

Results

Class A

Gravidas Group: The 6 patients, in whom we could get a function profile, did not show any evidence of GN progression during the period 'before'. In the period 'after' 2 cases (cases 11 and 12) showed an important deterioration (decrease of 50% or more) of renal function (No. 11 is today in ESRD).

Control Group: 2 patients (cases 1 and 4) showed functional deterioration of a similar degree (they are now transplanted and in RDT, respectively). As to the mean slope ($b \cdot 10^3$) of progression rate, the difference between the 'after' group (−1.872) and the control group (−1.571) was not statistically significant.

Class B

Gravidas Group: No significant change in the period 'before'; important deterioration in 1 case (case 3) in the period 'after'.

Control Group: No change as in gravidas in the period 'after'.

Class C

Gravidas Group: We have data for 'before' only in 6 patients who did not show any evidence of worsening renal function. In the period 'after', 6 of 8 cases showed a deterioration of renal function (fig. 1), very important in cases 1, 2 and 7 (No. 1 is now in ESRD).

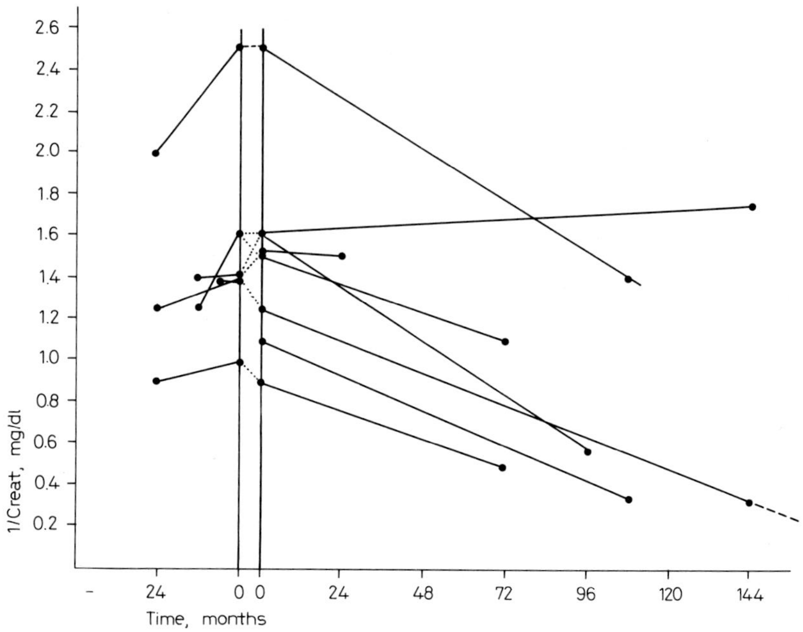

a

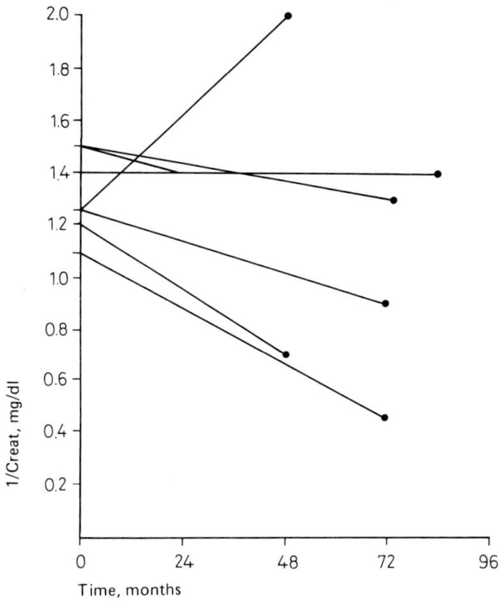

b

Fig. 1. Reciprocal of serum creatinine concentration (1/Creat) versus time in class C patients (focal segmental glomerulosclerosis). Behavior of reciprocal serum creatinine in gravidas group before and after pregnancy (*a*) and in the control group (*b*).

Control Group: In 1 patient (case 2) we observed a worsening to the same degree as in the 3 pregnant cases mentioned (fig. 1). The mean slopes of progression rate were different between the 'after' group (−4.728) and the control group (−2.173), but the difference was not statistically significant.

Class D

Gravidas Group: Case 2, who did not show any change during the period 'before' (60 months), had a marked deterioration of renal function in the period 'after' (24 months). Case 5 also worsened and progressed to ESRD.

Control Group: We did not observe any worsening of renal function.

Discussion

In this study on 29 primary glomerulonephritides who underwent pregnancy, we restricted our attention to the influence of gestation on the course of the kidney disease.

Review of the literature does not allow firm conclusions. Some investigators indeed believe that pregnancy does not adversely affect the natural course of GN [1, 2]; some others, in contrast, maintain that pregnancy often leads to a deterioration of renal function [3] and to a worsening of morphologic lesions [4].

One of the diffuculties in assessing the influence of pregnancy on the course of GN is that only small numbers of patients with any particular form of glomerular disease, as defined by histological examination, are included in most series. Another one is that the choice of the outcome of the disease as a parameter of evaluation of the course is often deceptive. The outcome would indeed have to be taken into account only after a period roughly equivalent in all patients. Cases with very different follow-up durations could hardly be compared to each other as regards outcome. For these reasons we also selected the deterioration rate of renal function as a parameter giving better evidence of the worsening effect of pregnancy on the course of GN.

To make an intra-patient comparison, we distinguished progression rates in the periods before and after pregnancy, but in the group 'before'

Table I. Reciprocal of serum creatinine concentration (l/Creat) at the beginning and end of the period before pregnancy or follow-up and at the beginning and end of the period pregnancy

Patient	A	B	C	D	E	F	$b^* \times 10^3$ before	$b^* \times 10^3$ after
Class A (Berger's disease)								
Gravidas group								
1 S.A.	1.33	1.00	60	0.88	1.00	60	– 5.5	2
2 C.L.		1.25		1.25	1.10	60		– 2.5
3 C.A.		1.10		1.25	1.00	156		– 1.60
4 D.C.		1.10		1.25	1.10	132		– 1.14
5 S.T.		1.25		1.33	0.90	72		– 5.97
6 R.I.		1.40		1.40	1.40	60		0
7 L.R.		1.25		1.33	1.25	60		– 1.33
8 O.M.	1.40	1.10	60	1.60	1.00	84	– 5	– 7.14
9 S.A.	1.00	1.40	60	1.40	1.40	12	6.67	0
10 P.G.	1.10	0.90	24	0.90	0.83	84	– 8.33	2.62
11 M.G.		1.00		1.00	0.30	132		– 5.30
12 C.G.	1.40	1.17	24	1.25	0.66	216	– 9.58	– 2.73
13 M.B.	1.40	1.60	60	1.33	1.12	168	3.33	– 1.25
Mean slope ($b \times 10^3$)							– 3.068 ± 0.56	– 1.872 ± 3.49
Control group								
1 C.D.	1.25	0.20				109		– 9.63
2 T.R.	1.60	1.40				84		– 2.38
3 M.A.	1.10	1.10				72	0	
4 C.I.	1.10	0.10				96		–10.42
5 D.A.	1.40	1.00				96		– 4.17
6 C.A.	1.25	1.10				84		– 1.79
7 B.R.	1.10	1.00				72		– 1.39
8 M.L.	1.40	1.40				72		0
9 J.G.	1.40	1.40				60		0
10 S.T.	2.00	2.00				24		0
11 B.A.	0.80	1.40				48		12.5
Mean slope ($b \times 10^3$)								1.571 ± 5.71

For explanations see p. 188.

Table I. (continued)

Patient	A	B	C	D	E	F	$b^* \times 10^3$	
							before	after
Class B (membranous glomerulonephritis)								
Gravidas group								
1 N.F.	1.00	1.00	12	1.00	0.83	24	0	– 7.08
2 P.G.	1.60	1.30	24	1.60	0.87	24	–12.5	–30.41
3 C.M.	1.20	1.00	24	1.00	0.27	120	–12	– 6.08
Mean slope ($b \times 10^3$)							– 8.16	–14.52
							± 7.07	± 13.76
Control group								
1 P.M.	1.10	1.40				120		2.5
2 G.L.	1.60	0.85				60		– 1.25
3 S.A.	1.10	1.53				84		5.12
Mean slope ($b \times 10^3$)								2.12
								± 3.2
Class C (focal segmental glomerulosclerosis)								
Gravidas group								
1 B.M.	1.25	1.40	24	1.25	0.16	288	6.25	
2 U.M.	1.25	1.60	12	1.60	0.57	96	29.17	
3 T.E.	0.90	1.00	24	0.90	0.50	72		
4 L.A.	1.40	1.40	12	1.53	1.50	24	0	– 1.15
5 C.F.	2.00	2.50	24	2.50	1.40	108	20.83	
6 L.N.	1.40	1.40	12	1.60	1.75	144	0	1.04
7 O.R.				1.10	0.35	108		– 6.94
8 C.A.		1.60		1.53	1.10	72		– 5.97
Mean slope ($b \times 10^3$)							11.25	– 3.25
							± 13.14	± 3.82
Control group								
1 M.O.	1.20	0.70				48		–10.42
2 C.G.	1.10	0.48				72		– 8.61
3 T.P.	1.25	0.90				72		– 4.86
4 P.M.	1.40	1.40				84		0
5 M.L.	1.50	1.40				24		– 4.17
6 P.O.	1.25	2.00				48		1.63
7 C.M.	1.50	1.30				72		– 2.78
Mean slope ($b \times 10^3$)								– 4.17
								± 4.32

For explanations see p. 188.

Table I. (continued)

Patient	A	B	C	D	E	F	b* × 10³ before	b* × 10³ after
Class D (membranoproliferative glomerulonephritis)								
Gravidas group								
1 C.A.		1.40		1.60	1.12	84		– 5.71
2 S.B.	1.40	1.33	60	1.60	0.58	24	– 1.17	–42.5
3 L.P.		1.60		1.40	1.10	180		– 1.67
4 E.L.		1.60		1.40	1.13	24		–11.25
5 R.L.				1.00	0.15	60		–14.17
Mean slope (b × 10³)							– 1.17	–15.06
							+ 0	± 16.08
Control group								
1 C.G.	1.10	1.40				60		5
2 S.L.	1.10	1.60				12		41.67
Mean slope (b × 10³)								23.34
								± 25.93

A = 1/Creat (mg/dl) at the beginning of the period before pregnancy or at the beginning of the follow-up.
B = 1/Creat (mg/dl) at the end of the period before pregnancy or at the end of follow-up.
C = Time interval (months) before pregnancy.
D = 1/Creat (mg/dl) at the beginning of the period after pregnancy.
E = 1/Creat (mg/dl) at the end of the period after pregnancy.
F = Time interval (months) after pregnancy or at the end of follow-up.
*b is the regression coefficient calculated by the equation: $y = a + bx$.

we observed no deterioration at all (Berger's disease) or only an unimportant one (GNM, GNMP, FSGS), so that all the cases reached pregnancy with renal function still in the normal range. The follow-up of the group 'before' was shorter than the 'after' one in classes A, B and C (44, 20 and 17 as regards 99, 56 and 114 months), while the follow-up of the control group was better matched with the 'after' group in these classes (74, 70 and 60, respectively). We do not think that the different follow-up durations could explain the discrepancy between the groups 'before' and 'after' as to the progression rate.

There has also been a remarkable difference in the slope of progression rate between the 'after' group and the control group in classes B, C and D, but a measure of the statistical significance could not be done because of the low degree of freedom in classes B and D.

As far as the outcome is concerned the difference was very important. 8 of 29 cases in the whole 'after' group showed severe deterioration of renal function (decrease of 1/Creat to 50% or less of the starting level) versus 3 of 23 cases of the control group. Among the former, 2 patients are today in ESRD and 1 in RDT; among the latter, 1 is in RDT, and 1 is transplanted.

Some authors [2] raised the objection that a long interval may question the connection between pregnancy and the outcome of GN, and claimed that only a temporal relationship between the former and the onset of renal failure might suggest a negative influence of the pregnancy. In all our cases, in whom a deterioration of renal function was observed after pregnancy, salient or trivial increases of serum creatinine concentration appeared quite early and fitted in quite well with the curve of progression.

In contrast with some data in the literature our findings seem to suggest that pregnancy adversely affects the progression rate and outcome of FSGS and MPGN, while there is no evidence of an effect on the course of Berger's disease.

References

1 Lindheimer, M.D.; Katz, A.I.: Kidney function and disease in pregnancy, (Lea & Febiger, Philadelphia, pp. 146–187 1977).

2 Katz, A.I.; Davison, J.M.; Hayslett, J.P.; Singson, E.; Lindheimer, M.D.: Pregnancy in women with kidney disease. Kidney int. *18*: 192–206 (1980).

3 Kincaid-Smith, P.; Fairley, K.F.: The differential diagnosis between preeclamptic toxemia and glomerulonephritis in patients with proteinuria during pregnancy; in Lindheimer, Kath, Zuspan, Hypertension in pregnancy, pp. 157–167 (Wiley, New York 1976).

4 Kincaid-Smith, P.; Whitworth, J.A.; Fairley, K.F.: Mesangial IgA nephropathy in pregnancy. Clin. exp. Hypertens. *2*: 821–838 (1980).

5 Rutherford, W.E.; Blondin, J.; Miller, J.P.; Greenwalt, A.S.; Vavra, J.D.: Chronic progressive renal disease: rate of change of serum creatinine concentration. Kidney int. *2*: 62–70 (1977).

C. Rovati, MD, Divisione di Nefrologia e Dialisi, Ospedale Niguarda Cà Granda, Piazza Ospedale Maggiore 3, I-20162 Milano (Italy)

Contr. Nephrol., vol. 37, pp. 190–193 (Karger, Basel 1984)

Control Studies of Women with Preeclampsia and Urinary Tract Infection in Pregnancy

Richard Schmicker, Gisela Vogel, Horst Klinkmann

Department of Internal Medicine, Wilhelm Pieck University, Rostock, GDR

Introduction

Preeclampsia may be considered as the most frequent complication of pregnancy. The frequency of preeclampsia differs depending on the geographical area and according to data in the literature it varies between 5 and 20% [3]. Essential preeclampsia will frequently occur in nulliparas. In multiparas, however, symptoms of preeclampsia are frequently due to preexisting vascular and renal diseases [1, 2].

Another important factor is the urinary tract infection (UTI) in pregnancy. It is often stated that bacteriuria is more common during pregnancy. However, numerous studies of pregnant women show that the incidence of bacteriuria is within the range known to exist in nonpregnant women of the same age. But it is important to know that about 40% of pregnant women with bacteriuria will develop symptomatic UTI if untreated [4]. The present investigation is aimed at examining the various causes of preeclampsia and UTI in pregnancy

Patients

Follow-up examinations were made in the preeclampsia dispensary of our department in 264 women affected with symptoms of preeclampsia during their pregnancy and in 60 women affected with UTI during their pregnancy. Control examinations began 3 months after delivery. The proposal made by the Committee on Terminology of the American College of Obstetricians and Gynecologists (ACOG) was used for classification.

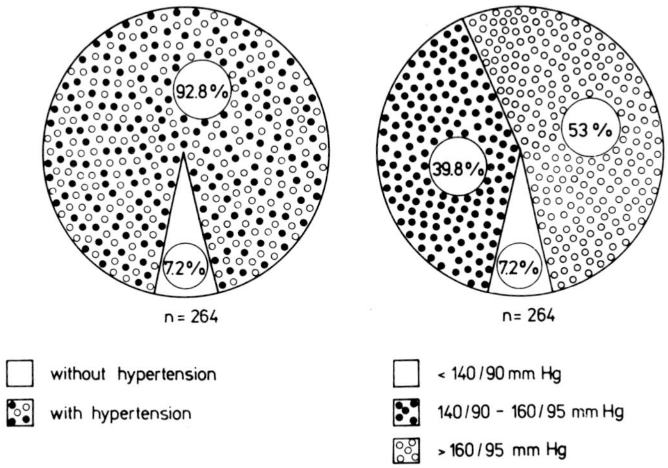

Fig. 1. Frequency of hypertension in the pregnancy of women with preeclampsia.

Results

In the total of 264 women affected with symptoms of preeclampsia 30 (11.4%) could be identified to have had hypertension in their anamnesis, and 76 (28.8%) of them to have had a UTI. Hypertension as the most important symptom of preeclampsia was calculated from 140/90mm Hg according to the definition of hypertension for preeclampsia. The frequency of hypertension in the pregnancy of women with preeclampsia can be seen in figure 1. In accordance with the definition mentioned, 92.8% (n = 245) of women had hypertension. Blood pressure was above 160/95mm Hg in 53% (n = 140) of them. As early as beginning from the 20th week of pregnancy an increased blood pressure could be detected in 15.9% (n = 39) from a total of 245 pregnant women with hypertension, whereas it occurred in 75.1% (n = 184) after the 20th week of pregnancy or in 9% (n = 22) during parturition.

Table I shows the various causes of preeclampsia. These diagnoses were performed during pregnancy. Essential preeclampsia could be diagnosed in 16.3% (n = 43). From the total of 264 women who had had symptoms of preeclampsia during pregnancy and who were sent to control examinations to our preeclampsia dispensary there were 16 (6.1%) who did not appear for specialized diagnostics so that no final diagnosis could be made. In the group of UTI during pregnancy this percentage amounted to 16.7% (n = 10).

Table I. Diagnoses during pregnancy in 264 women with preeclampsia

	%	n
Essential preeclampsia	16.3	43
Eclampsia	0.8	2
Secondary preeclampsia	38.6	102
Transitory hypertension	7.6	20
Chronic hypertension	29.5	78
Nonhypertensive preeclampsia	7.2	19

Table II. Diagnoses 3 months after delivery in 264 women with preeclampsia

	%	n
Normal findings	20.1	53
Chronic UTI	45.8	121
Chronic glomerulonephritis	1.5	4
Essential hypertension	26.5	70
No final diagnosis	6.1	16

Table II illustrates the findings of control investigations performed 3 months after delivery in women with preeclampsia. There were no pathological results in 20.1% (n = 53) of these checked female patients. Among these 53 women essential preeclampsia during pregnancy could be diagnosed in 30 cases, transitory hypertension in 14 cases, and non hypertensive preeclampsia in 8 cases. In nearly all cases secondary preeclampsia or chronic hypertension was observed during pregnancy in those women with chronic UTI and essential hypertension as the final diagnosis after delivery. These results emphasize the significance of preexcisting vascular and renal diseases for the development of symptoms of preeclampsia. Chronic UTI could be diagnosed in our control studies in 38.5% of 78 cases with chronic hypertension in pregnancy.

In 45 cases of the 60 women with UTI during pregnancy chronic UTI could be found by control investigations 3 months after delivery. In these cases an acute exacerbation of the chronic UTI was the cause of symptoms during pregnancy.

Conclusions

Because of the high percentage of preexisting vascular and renal diseases in women with preeclampsia all patients with symptoms of preeclampsia are required to be checked up after delivery. Even those women with UTI during pregnancy should be diagnosed nephrologically.

The value of control examinations made in the 324 women consists in the diagnosis and early therapy of preexisting vascular and renal diseases and in improving the prognosis for mother and fetus in case of a new pregnancy.

References

1 Chesley, L.C.: Hypertension in pregnancy: definitions, familial factor, and remote prognosis. Kidney int. *18*: 234–240 (1980).

2 Katz, A.I.; Davison, J.M.; Hayslett, J.P.; Singson, E.; Lindheimer, M.D.: Pregnancy in women with kidney disease. Kidney int. *18*: 192–206 (1980).

3 Kyank, H.: Präeklampsie – Eklampsie: in Kyank, Gülzow, Erkrankungen während der Schwangerschaft. pp. 211–227 (Thieme, Leipzig 1972).

4 Petri, E.; Klippel, K.F.: Pyelonephritis und Schwangerschaft. Nieren-Hochdruckkrankheiten *9*: 53–59 (1980).

Doz. Dr. R. Schmicker, Klinik für Innere Medizin, Wilhelm-Pieck-Universität, Ernst-Heydemann-Strasse, DDR-2500 Rostock (GDR)

Subject Index